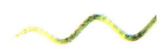

Grow Your Own Spirulina Superfood

a simple guide

by
Dr. Aaron Wolf Baum
of AlgaeLab LLC
http://algaelab.org

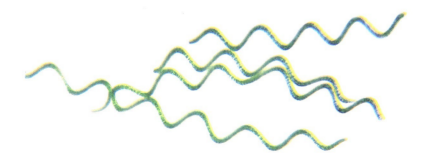

copyright © 2013 by AlgaeLab LLC

Acknowledgements:

I humbly acknowledge the essential assistance of Jean-Paul Jourdan and the good folks at Antenna (whom I have not yet had the pleasure of meeting), Hendrik van Poederooijen of the Simplicity spirulina farm, Daniel Fleischer, John Benemann, everyone who has helped me and AlgaeLab.org to reach this point, and my incomparable partner in life, Massey Burke.

Important statement about liability, PLEASE READ:

While I have no reason to think that there is any danger involved in growing and consuming spirulina that you grow yourself, this is a new process which we are still learning about, and hazards to your health cannot be ruled out, even if you do follow our instructions.

To make this process as safe as possible, follow these instructions TO THE LETTER and do not eat your spirulina if pH is low (<10), color is off (anything but deep blue-green), or you have any other reason to think that anything might be amiss with your culture. I also strongly recommend getting a microscope and monitoring your culture to make sure that no other algae (or other organisms) are growing there.

Please READ THE INSTRUCTIONS CAREFULLY, use common sense, and take any additonal precautions that might be appropriate for your situation, medical conditions, etc.

Table of Contents

Introduction 1

Section 1: Frequently Asked Questions 3

Section 2: Getting Started 13

Section 3: Growing Your Spirulina 16

Section 4: Harvesting Your Spirulina 25

Section 5: Culture Maintenance 37

Section 6: Alternative Harvest Techniques 39

Section 7: Expanding Your Setup 40

Section 8: Spirulina Growing Tips 48

Section 9: For More Information	54
Troubleshooting Guide	55
Appendix A: *Nutrient Mix Recipes*	64
Appendix B: *Growing Up From a Test Tube*	67

Introduction

When I first began my work in algae, seven rich and wonderful years ago, I looked everywhere for helpful material, but found only Ph.D.-level tomes, and sketchy, contradictory information on the Internet. I read the Ph.D.-level material, went to algae conferences, talked to professors and professionals, and gathered every bit of algae information I could find. Then I began growing it myself, and getting involved in professional algae projects. In the absence of basic, well-organized information, I progressed through trial and error, constant foraging for information among experts and scientific literature, and, sometimes, forehead-slapping discoveries. In the process, I became a scientist in the NASA OMEGA algae biofuel project, and discovered the many benefits of growing my own Spirulina at home, but still I found no good introduction into the world of algae farming for non-scientist types. After years of teaching workshops, and developing and selling home-grow kits, I have developed this this book as the next step of my effort to provide algae farming information to a wide audience, and give everyone a chance to join this amazing revolution in agriculture.

I hope you'll join me in this fun and rewarding algae adventure!

Dr. Aaron Wolf Baum,
February 2013

Have a look at my Spirulina window farm...

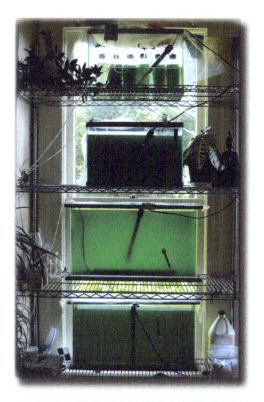

Figure 1: One of my Spirulina set-ups.

Every day, I flip a switch and a little pump starts the process of gathering today's harvest, passing green algae culture from one of my tanks through the harvest cloth. The water goes back into the tank; the microscopic algae spirals are caught on the cloth and form a rich dark blue-green paste packed with concentrated nutritional goodness. I spoon it into a shake, mix it with soup or salad dressing, put it in the fridge for later, or freeze it. It is easy to combine with food because of its minimal taste and creamy texture, unlike the funky-tasting store-bought powders. The only way to get it is by growing it myself. The bubbling blue-green culture has a cool, futuristic look to it, and once visitors understand what it does, they often want to start growing it themselves...

I started with a few tanks in a window (see above), but wanting more and more of that precious blue-green stuff, I am moving outside, where I can capture more light and create more growth. Soon I'll create an even larger growth pond in a greenhouse, and start selling Spirulina in my local farmers' market... It's a new, high-yield kind of farming that's rewarding, fun, and surprisingly easy, and I'd love to share how it works with you...

Shall we get started?

Section 1: Frequently-Asked Questions

Let's start with the most commonly-asked questions about algae and Spirulina:

What are Algae?

Almost everyone has seen green stuff growing in pools, ponds, or bird baths, but few people know much about what that stuff really is. **Algae – to be more specific, micro-algae – are microscopic plants that live floating in water.** Although you need a microscope to see them individually, their numbers are often so great that they make large bodies of water – even oceans – green.

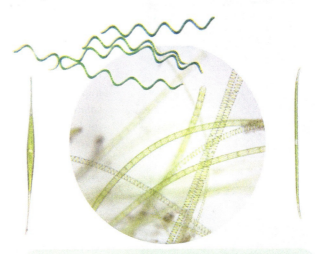

Figure 2: A few microscopic pictures of algae. To the left and right, freshwater diatoms. Spirulina colonies hover above. Magnifaction is 400x.

Why Algae?

Because algae are amazing, and everyone should know about what they can do! They enable a new kind of agriculture that can be done almost anywhere. Algae grow in boiling hot springs and antarctic snows, and in acidic, basic, and saline water in which no other creatures can live. Algae can be farmed on deserts (with just a little water!), in industrial wastes, and on the surface of the ocean. *No soil or farmland is required.*

Algae are also incredible productive, even in small spaces. Because algae cells live floating in a nutrient broth (called the "growth medium"), they don't need to rely on a nutrient delivery system, as plants do; and unlike plants they do not have to produce roots, leaves, stalks, or stems – they just make more of themselves, constantly... On a good day, algae can double their numbers up to three times – this means that if you start the day with one pound of algae, you end the day with as much as eight pounds! Algae can also convert 10-25x more of their bodies into desirable products – for example, many algae can be 50+% oil, versus 2-3% for soybeans and other typical oil crops currently used for oil. Together, these traits mean that *algae can produce more than 100x as much product per acre as compared to conventional land crops.*

They can produce a vast array of products, from antioxidants to biodiesel, protein to chemical precursors, omega-3 fatty acids, alcohol, nano-structured glass, and many others, with new ones being discovered all the time. This is due to the vast diversity of algae, which exceeds that of all animals, plants, and fungi combined.

Algae can be grown using minimal resources. Because an algae pond or tank is inherently self-contained, water and nutrients do not pass into the soil, and evaporation is much less than in land plants. Algae can derive their nutrients from wastewater and combustion exhaust, producing cleaner water and air. Nutrients can be recycled from harvested algae after the desired products have been extracted. For these reasons, they can be grown with minimal or even positive impact on the natural environment.

And the potential of algae farming is truly vast. Because it is so productive, and because you can grow it anywhere, algae's economic potential exceeds that of all of agriculture existing today. In the last several years, dozens of new algae companies have plunged hundreds of millions of dollars[1] into research and development – and by reading this book you can join in!

---

[1] For example, check out algae companies such as Aurora Algae, Algenol, Sapphire Energy, Solix Biofuels, and projects such as the NASA OMEGA project.

Is Algae Farming New?

Why haven't most people heard of algae farming before? Algae have been around for billions of years, and have been eaten by humans for hundreds if not thousands of years,[2] but intentional algae farming is relatively new. Though people have been growing land crops for about ten thousand years, the first large-scale algae farms were created only about sixty years ago. It's no wonder that few people have even heard of algae farming! This is also why so much of what is happening in the algae world is research and development; even so, there is much that DIY-ers can do, and now is a great opportunity to get in on the ground floor, while this field is still emerging.

Why Spirulina?

There are at least 30,000 known species of algae, and more are being discovered all the time. Only a few have been grown commercially, though hundreds are under research for future farming scenarios. Enthusiasts new to algae often want to grow many different species; in particular, many have heard of algae biofuels.

A word about growing food versus fuel:
The last few years, the media has been ahum with the promise of algae biofuels. I believe in this promise, and have worked on a number of algae biofuel projects, including the NASA OMEGA project. Many DIY-ers have contacted me about the possibility of producing biofuel from algae on small farms, etc. I certainly encourage amateur innovators in the field, but it is important to understand that, as our cars use far more energy than our bodies, it takes roughly one acre of algae pond (plus oil-extracting and biodiesel conversion gear) to produce enough fuel to power even a fuel-efficient car every day. This is why I generally direct amateur growers toward Spirulina and other food algae over biofuel. Many advances in algaculture technology are being made, and may greatly improve the prospect for amateur algae biofuel in the future.

While I try to help all budding algae farmers, **I always recommend that beginners start with Spirulina. This is for five basic reasons: it is easy to grow, amazingly good for you, easy to harvest, easy to use, and produces a high-value product that cannot be obtained in any other way.** I don't know of any other algae species that combines these virtues, or that has been so thoroughly proven-out as a valuable health

---

[2] Aztecs ate Spirulina harvested from natural soda lakes in Mexico for several hundred years, and tribes in Chad have a long-standing tradition of harvesting, selling, and preparing natural Spirulina (*"dihe"*) into a soup.

supplement. Spirulina is certainly the best way to start algae farming, and is a highly worthwhile crop in any case — which is why I wrote this book!

Here are the five reasons in more detail:

1. Spirulina is easy (and safe) to grow.

As anyone who has left a swimming pool or other body of water unattended knows, it is not difficult to grow some kind of green stuff in any body of water exposed to sunlight. But this is actually the problem: it is generally challenging to grow just one species of algae, as the nutrients put into the water to grow the desired species may also allow undesired, contaminating species of algae to multiply. As you can probably imagine, pulling out billions of microscopic weeds is rather tricky! Factor in the fact that many wild algae species can make nasty toxins, and you've got the ingredients for some serious headaches.

This is where Spirulina's first superpower comes into play. Spirulina is an alkaliphile, meaning that it loves to grow in extremely alkaline water, at pH values (10+)[3] that exclude almost all other forms of life. In the wild, Spirulina grows in natural soda lakes, where native peoples (Aztecs in Mexico, and various tribes in Africa) have been harvesting and eating it for hundreds of years, taking advantage of the lack of toxic algae in these lakes to obtain this highly nutritious food source. What this means for the amateur algae grower is that, as long as you keep the pH above 10, you can generally maintain a pure culture if you maintain basic precautions – covering the tank carefully, and washing your hands before working with your algae. Spirulina are one of the few types of algae that can be grown outdoors in open ponds relatively safely, though at these larger scales close monitoring is important, as contamination is likely if the pH ever drops. pH testing is an integral part of growing Spirulina.

An important note about "blue-green algae" products: you may have seen "blue-green algae" health products in stores, advertising all sorts of health benefits. I do not recommend the consumption of these products, as they are wild-harvested algae, with a significant risk of contamination by toxin-producing algae. While Spirulina is a type of blue-green algae, it is very different in that it is grown under controlled conditions, in an alkaline medium that excludes toxic algae. Also, the safety of eating Spirulina has been demonstrated both by hundreds of studies on animals and people,[4] and by the long history of Spirulina consumption by pre-industrial people. No other type of algae has been studied as much both for its benefits (see below) and its safety.

---

3   pH is a measurement of the acidity or basicity of a solution; see the section on "pH and How to Measure It" for more details.

4   For example, see: *Spirulina in Human Nutrition and Health*, M.E. Gershwin and A. Belay eds., CRC Press, 2008.

2. Spirulina is amazingly good for you.

Why are health conscious folks so nutty for Spirulina? Spirulina cells have several unusual properties that make them a unique food supplement that can significantly enhance your health. First off, unlike most plants, which are about 90% indigestible cellulose, Spirulina does not have a cell wall or any other indigestible components. Spirulina completely dissolves when you eat it, and has almost no bulk, making it a a super-concentrated, highly available nutrient source, which enhances the nutrition of any food eaten with it. Because our vitality depends on the nutrients we can extract from the food that we have in our system – and we can only fit so much inside our bodies – the nutrient density of the food we eat determines (in part) whether we feel like taking care of business, or taking a nap. By adding a little Spirulina to our diet – to every meal if possible – we can increase the availabilty of the building blocks our body uses to feed and heal itself.

Spirulina is jammed with healthful stuff. It about 65% complete protein — twice the density of beef or sushi — and the remainder is anti-oxidants, essential omega-3 fatty acids, and other healthful things. Since blue-green algae like Spirulina are evolutionarily distant from just about every other food that we eat (having split from the line that led to green plants approximately a billion years ago), they are rich in nutritional substances that cannot be found in other foods, including the brilliant blue pigments phycocyanin and allophycocyanin, which are powerful antioxidants, and GLA, which is a potent anti-inflammatory.[5] Spirulina has been studied far more than any other sort of algae both for its lack of negative effects, and for its many positive effects. Clinical studies, both in animals and in humans, have shown dramatic benefits for improving stamina, balancing the immune system, leveling blood sugar, reducing blood cholesterol, increasing beneficial bacteria in the gut, and protection against toxins, as well as anti-inflammatory, anti-viral, and anti-cancer properties.[6]

There are other sound reasons to add Spirulina to you diet. Eating "close to the earth" – i.e. eating plants rather than animals – is a good idea in general, as many toxins tend to get concentrated in the bodies of animals from their diet of plants. **One of the great benefits of growing your own Spirulina is the ability to completely control the whole food production process, to ensure that the food you produce is as pure as possible.** This is in contrast to conventional farming — including Spirulina farming — which is highly exposed to airborne pollutants, bird feces, etc. **As Spirulina is the only non-animal source of concentrated complete**

---

5 GLA (gamma linolenic acid) can be found in other foods, such as Evening Primrose oil, but Spirulina has the most of any food.

6 For a review of such studies, see *Spirulina in Human Nutrition and Health*, M.E. Gershwin and A. Belay eds., CRC Press, 2008.

protein, it can enable a very clean vegan diet. As a highly active 200-pound man I never thought I could eat vegan until I started including Spirulina in my diet, which makes vegetables, fruits, and grains much more satisfying. Having such a clean diet is really eye-opening; my skin has acquired a new glow.

I started taking Spirulina in large doses all at once – 15+ grams a day – while keeping everything else in my (otherwise balanced and healthy) diet constant, to see if I could isolate the effects it had on me. Most noticeable was a distinct improvement in stamina; if I work hard, I still get tired, but after a moment's rest I am back in the game. I also found that helped a lot to stabilize my blood sugar, eliminating spikes and valleys to even out my mood, which makes me a much happier person. This result is consistent with clinical studies that show a large reduction (up to 50%) in the glycemic index of foods eaten with even a small amount (2.5%) of Spirulina.[7] I also find that taking Spirulina speeds recovery from workouts and wound healing. I have since upped my intake to 20 grams a day (3 heaping tablespoons of the powder, or 6 of the fresh stuff), and experienced even more benefits. When I have taken even more (up to 30 grams) I just feel better, but it's just challenging to include that much in my diet![8]

3. Spirulina is easy to harvest.
Even if an algae culture seems thick and green, it's usually not more than about 1 gram of non-water biomass per liter of water; in other words, about 99.9% water. In order to actually use your algae, you'll need to somehow get them out of the water (you can't drink the culture directly, as it is full of plant nutrients are not meant to be consumed in large quantities). Since algae cells are microscopic, this can be an interesting challenge! Most forms of algae require fairly complex equipment to separate them from the medium they are growing in; the most common way is by using a centrifuge, an expensive and rather technical piece of equipment (though small ones are highly useful in any well equipped algae lab!).

Once again, Spirulina neatly fixes this problem for us, this time with its shape, a corkscrew spiral which lends itself to simple filtration using easily-obtained screen printing fabric. Just pour the culture through the cloth, and the algae are caught on top, while the water passes right through... the shape of the spiral means that the accumulating algae form a matrix that has many pores, allowing the water to pass through even as the algae accumulate. This is in contrast to typical small-

---

7   See "Glycemic Index of Spirulina-Supplemented Meals", U. Iyer, S. Deshmukh, and U. Mani, Int. J. Diab. Dev. Countries (1999), Vol. 19; and "Antidiabetic Property of Spirulina", A. Layam and C. L. K. Reddy, Diabetologia Croatica 35-2, 2006.

8   Most studies of the benefits of Spirulina are done using doses between 1 and 10 grams. I recommend consulting a physician if you plan to eat more than that. Experts recommend eating no more than 50 grams a day in any case.

cell algae, which pass right through even the finest fabric, and even if you do have small enough pores the cells quickly form an impenetrable mass that slows the filtering process to a crawl.

4. Spirulina is easy to use.

In most forms of algae farming, after the algae have been extracted from the water, the cells must be broken open, and the desired products extracted. If you've heard of Spirulina you've probably heard of Chlorella, another form of algae that also has positive health properties; its cells, though, are very small, round, and have an exceedingly tough outer wall. The cell wall is so physically and chemically tough that they can pass right through your digestive tract unharmed. As such, they are difficult to harvest, and the cell wall must be ruptured if we are to get any nutrients from them whatsoever; this takes additional work and extra equipment.

Utilizing freshly harvested Spirulina couldn't be easier – pop it in your smoothie, salad dressing, or soup, or just pop it in your mouth! Have a look at our Recipes (Section 11) for more ideas...

5. Spirulina produces a high-value product that cannot be obtained any other way. Spirulina provides a much better return on the money and time you invest in its growth than practically any other crop, including other types of algae. For example, compare the value of algae biofuels, simply on a dollar basis. At $4.50/gallon, diesel fuel is worth $0.65/pound, compared to Spirulina, which sells for $20/pound or more... And fresh Spirulina is a better product than the powdered stuff, as it has much better texture and taste, making it much easier to combine with food. Furthermore, if you grow it yourself you can be sure of its purity and quality. At this time, there are no commercial sources I know of for fresh Spirulina.

And then there is the difference in health benefits between eating fresh Spirulina versus packaged powder. All studies of the health benefits of Spirulina have been on the powdered stuff, as it is much easier to obtain. It stands to reason, though, that the fresh version of such a highly perishable food would have superior properties, and this is my experience, having eaten both. Purveyors of the powder claim they take every precaution to preserve the nutritional properties of the algae, but what would you rather eat, a fresh blueberry, or a powdered blueberry? Grow it yourself and see!

Is Algae Farming For Me?

So, should you try your hand at algae farming? Perhaps you have killed some house plants in your past and are a little shy about trying to raise any more green stuff. In many ways, though, growing Spirulina is easier than other kinds of plants; it certainly requires a lot less space (just one sunny window will do), and is more rewarding. Here are quick answers to the six main questions prospective algae farmers always ask me. The rest of the book attempts to expand on these answers...

What Do I Need to Start Algae Farming?

Maybe a lot less than you think:

1. A sunny spot. Best is a south-facing window without shading trees, buildings, etc., or a spot outside with good southern exposure. Partly shaded, east- or west-facing windows will also do. Artificial lighting can also be used.

2. A tank or other container for the algae. This can be as simple as a fish tank or pond.

3. Water. Almost any potable water source can be used to grow algae — see "Using the Right Water", p. 20 below.

4. Nutrients. Combine a few food-grade fertilizers according to Appendix A, or buy pre-formulated mixes for Spirulina at AlgaeLab.org.

5. Live algae starter. You can order starter culture from AlgaeLab.org, or an algae culture library (see Appendix B).

A few additional items may be helpful, see the list in the Getting Started section below.

Will It Smell?

Perhaps you or someone you know has been near a stagnant algae bloom in the wild which is decomposing. This can smell really bad; but living, healthy algae cultures don't smell at all. Unless you leave it unattended for months, or put something in your tank that doesn't belong, this will not be a concern. **A living algae culture actually freshens the room it is in**, by producing oxygen and eliminating carbon dioxide and other pollutants.

How Much Harvest Will I Get?

Since Spirulina is probably the easiest and most rewarding species for beginners, let's use that as an example. If the culture is properly set up and fed, its output will be determined by the amount of light striking the culture. What this means is that the amount of Spirulina you get will be equal to its area facing the sun, times the number of hours it spends in direct sunshine.[9] If you plan to use artificial illumination (see section 8 for more details about how best to do this), you can still use these numbers as a guide.[10]

While a clever system design can optimize the delivery of light to the algae, an average output of 25 dry weight grams per square meter per day[11] is about as high as can be sustainably produced under optimal conditions and lots of sun. For blue-green species such as Spirulina, 10 grams per square meter per day is what is typically attained under optimal conditions.

5 grams per day is a good amount to supplement a human diet, so 0.5 square meters (about 5.5 square feet) with excellent sun is enough to significantly improve the life of one person. This is a highly managable size for an algae farm, even if you have a full-time job, etc.

How Much Will It Cost?

At this time, a 10-gallon algae growth kit, with supplies for approximately a year, sells in the AlgaeLab.org store for $299. If you want to assemble a kit yourself, you can buy a one liter bottle of Spirulina starter culture for $69, and probably save a little money.

One such 10-gallon tank in a sunny window can produce about 12 grams of fresh Spirulina a day,[12] which translates to 10 pounds a year. Freshly-harvested Spirulina has far superior taste, texture, and nutrition to commercial powdered stuff, but cannot be bought commercially (yet!), so there's no sure way to judge its value, but if you say it's worth $25/lb, that gives a return of $250 per tank per year. If you

---

9 Mathematically inclined folk will point out that it is equal to these things times a proportionality constant...

10 For an artificially lit system, yield is proportional to the number of watts of light absorbed by the culture.

11 1 square meter is about 11 square feet.

12 Fresh Spirulina is about 75% water by weight, so this is equivalent to 3 grams per day dry weight.

buy a kit, then expand with a second tank (which will cost you about $50), after a year you'll have spent about $299, but produced algae worth $500; after two years, you'll have produced algae worth $1000 versus about $399 in... of course larger scale is where the economy truly kicks in.

How Much Time Does It Take?

Like any endeavor, growing algae can take as much time as you want to put into it, but a simple Spirulina tank takes very little work – about an hour of initial set-up, ten minutes or so for every harvest, and then cleaning the tank and/or changing out the medium every six months or so, which takes about 90 minutes. It's less work than a vegetable patch, with a higher-value product that you can't buy at the grocery store!

How Do I Get Started?

A great question, see the next chapter...

Section 2: Getting Started

A Little Terminology

Here are a few terms often used in algae farming, with which you should acquaint yourself:

Medium: A mixture of water and nutrients, intended to optimize the growth of algae. The plural is **media**.

Culture: Algae growing in their medium.

Inoculum: The "starter" culture used to seed a new culture.

Photobioreactor: A fancy name for an enclosed container used to grow algae.

Where to Put Your Algae Farm

The first thing to do is find a good spot for your growing set-up. The most important thing is to find a spot that gets as much SUN as possible; the more *direct* sunbeams that hit your tank, the more growth you will get. For indoor growth, your best bet is to put your tank in a south-facing window without buildings, trees, etc. that block direct sunlight. If you can grow outdoors, use a spot that gets as much direct sun as possible. As Spirulina like fairly high temperatures — 85-98 degrees Fahrenheit — outside the tropics you'll get best results growing outdoors in a greenhouse or other transparent enclosure.

When deciding how to support your algae tank, keep in mind that a full tank can be quite heavy; a full 10-gallon tank (holding 8.5 gallons) weighs about 75 pounds. A stainless steel rack (like the one in Figure 1) is a good solution, though most sturdy pieces of furniture will work.

You will also need to have a way to position a bucket next to the tank, lower than the tank if possible. If the lip of the bucket is 6" below the lip of the tank, this is about right. (See Section 6 for alternatives to bucket-wrangling...) Also keep in mind that there may be some spillage of your green liquid; put a waterproof layer over any carpets or not-wettable stuff in the potential "spill zone".

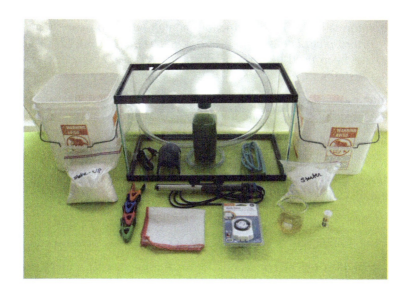

Figure 3: A complete AlgaeLab kit, plus tank, buckets, and beaker. Everything needed for your algae adventure!

Algae Farming Equipment

Once you have picked out your spot, here's what you'll need to grow your own Spirulina (see picture above).

Necessary Equipment

This is the gear that is needed to carry out the instructions in this book.

1. **An aquarium, or other transparent container to hold the culture.** 10 gallons is a good size to start with, and inexpensive 10-gallon aquariums (as shown in the pictures) work well. A key factor in choosing your container is the ability of light to reach every part of the culture; you don't want any part of the culture to be more than about 6 inches from a light source. This means that a tank one foot wide is OK, as long as it is transparent and getting some light on all sides. Also, when choosing your container, keep in mind that you will need to be able to clean it out thoroughly from time to time.

2. **A cover for your tank;** it doesn't need to be air-tight (and actually must allow the bubbling air to leave), but should keep out dust and other contamination.

3. **Live Spirulina.** You can order a liter bottle from AlgaeLab.org, or buy smaller amounts at higher cost from culture libraries (see Appendix B for culture li-

brary information). These instructions apply to the two main strains of Spirulina – *Arthrospira platensis* and *Arthrospira maxima* – as well as related strains that have been used for food production. We use, and sell, a well-proven *platensis* strain.

4. **Air pump** of a size appropriate for the tank; the smallest size works for a 10-gallon tank. Pick a quiet one if you're going to have it in your living space.
5. **Some aquarium air tubing**, enough to stretch from wherever you put the air pump to the bottom of your tank.
6. **Diffusers/bubblers/airstones** sufficient to generate bubbles around all the inside walls of the tank;
7. **4 or more clothespins** or other clips;
8. **¾"+ dia. Tubing**, 18-24" long, for harvest siphon (see harvest section below);
9. **pH strips or a pH meter** capable of measuring at least a range of 9.5-10.5 pH — the best strips are from pHydrion (see "pH, and How to Check It" on page 28 below).
10. **Harvest cloth screen** printing fabric with 40-50 micron openings (also called 300 mesh, or 120 thread);
11. **"Starter" and "Make-up" nutrient mixes** – see Appendix A at end of this document for recipes. Pre-mixed nutrients can be bought from AlgaeLab.org, and are provided with the kits.
12. **Tablespoon and teaspoon** measuring spoons.
13. **Two 5-gallon buckets**, for culture wrangling.

Optional Equipment

This is the gear that it is a very good idea to have, but not absolutely necessary.

1. **Aquarium heater**, capable of maintaining the tank at 80 degrees F or more. I recommend Eheim-Jager heaters, as they can be set to 94F or even higher. If your culture gets plenty of strong sunshine, and your house is not particularly cold, you may not need a heater. 100W is a good size for a 10-gallon tank.
2. **Aquarium thermometer**, to keep track of your culture's temperature. The most convenient type has a suction cup so it can be stuck where it is fully immersed in the culture and can be easily read.
3. **Plug timer**, to turn the heater off at night; this is a good idea if you're using a heater.
4. **A piece of white fabric**, big enough to shade your tank from direct sunshine. It should be as thin as possible without allowing actual rays to pass through

(i.e. diffuse light only).

5. **A water pump**, to make harvesting faster and easier. The smallest type of aquarium pump works well.
6. **A scale** for measuring out ingredients to make your own nutrient mixes. This should be accurate to 0.001 grams, i.e. one milligram.
7. **A microscope** for looking at your new friends, and making sure that they are the only critters in your tank! This should be at least 100x; you'll see more with 400x though. "Inverted" microscopes are easier, as cover slips are not needed; you'll need microscope slides in any case...

A full kit, with all the necessary components (except the tank and cover), plus heater, timer, and thermometer is available at AlgaeLab.org. See Figure 3. Although I will sometimes refer to these kits and the starter algae, as I designed them to make this process much easier, I have made sure everywhere to include enough information so that you can grow on your own, from scratch, using the information in this book.

Section 3: Growing Your Spirulina

Taking Care of the Spirulina Starter (Inoculum)

If you have a liter of culture from AlgaeLab.org, you can put it into your tank as soon as you have it set up and get going... if you are starting with a small test-tube from an algae culture library, you will need to grow it up to about a liter before taking this step. See Appendix B, "Growing Up from a Test Tube", for tips on how to do this.

When your bottle of starter Spirulina is being shipped or transported, it's obviously important to keep the lid on tight to keep it from spilling. But as soon as you can, put it in a spot that has plenty of light but no direct sunlight, remove the cap, and if you have a cotton ball or two, use them to fill the mouth of the bottle so it can breathe without becoming contaminated. If you don't have any cotton balls, just loosening the cap as much as possible is OK. If you have an air pump and a little air tubing (such as come with the kit), run bubbles through the culture to keep it mixed. If not, swirl it gently to re-suspend the algae (making a uniform green soup) as often as possible, at least once a day. This is also how to maintain a reserve culture, to re-start your culture if something goes wrong. Start the culture as described below as soon as possible; the algae can survive this way for weeks, sometimes even months, but they'll grow better if this period is kept to a minimum.

Setting Up the Growth Tank

To get set up, put your tank in its spot. Next you will set up the air pump and bubbler, and the heater, if you're using one.

Because the turbulence created by the bubbles will help prevent algae from clumping and sticking to the walls, it is best to **position the bubblers so that they are close to the walls**, and if possible all walls should have bubbles running past them. This also makes the bubbles more visible, adding to the "cool green bubbling stuff", mad scientist effect... A flexible bubble wand works well for this, as it can be run along the edge of the tank (see Figure 4); if you have a differently-shaped container, try to replicate this arrangement as well as you can. Attach the bubbler to the air pump, inserting the check valve (which should be included with the bubbler) into the line to prevent culture from running back into the air pump.[13] Blow into the check valve to make sure you're inserting it in the right direction, so that air can flow.

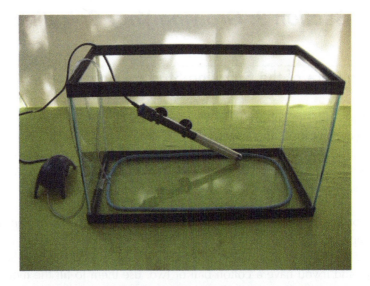

Figure 4: Initial tank set-up. Note position of heater and bubbler wand.

You are only going to fill the bottom quarter of the tank to start with, so you'll need

---

13 If you don't have a check valve, don't despair, the setup will work fine without it. It is just a precaution against an unlikely (though messy) event.

to **position the heater properly**. Attach the heater to the lower part of the side of the tank – making sure the hot part of the heater will be fully submerged. If the heater is "fully submersible" – it will say so on the package – put it close to the bottom, and horizontal. Otherwise, you'll need to fiddle with the angle a little to make sure the top (non-submersible) part is out of the water while the glass heater part is fully submerged.

> **An important note about electricity, water, and safety:**
> **Aquarium heaters can be dangerous!** Be sure to unplug them whenever they are out of the water, even for a short time, as they will heat up to temperatures that can burn the skin. Also, if you leave a heater on while out of water, and then put it in water, the glass may break. THIS IS A DANGEROUS SITUATION, as you now have bare electrical elements in water – someone could get shocked if they touch the water! Unplug the heater immediately, then deal with it. The heaters we use for the kit (Eheim-Jager) use thicker, stronger glass than most, and so are more resistant to breakage. And while we're at it, do I need to tell you to **be very careful about combining water and electricity in general**? Watch for dripping water going along power cords - keep plugs high so water can't drip into them, and set things up so that electrical devices like the air pump cannot be knocked into the tank!

Plug the heater into a plug timer. The Spirulina grow best when they are cool at night (up to a point, see the Temperature section on page 49), so set the timer to turn off the heater at dusk, and to turn on the heater two to three hours before dawn. If you are using grow lights, you will get maximum growth using 24-hour illumination and heating; if you do turn off the lights, turn off the heater as well.

A dilute culture, and especially one that is just being started, is more sensitive to light than a thick, mature culture. **Too much light can actually harm such a Spirulina culture**. For this reason, shade your culture initially from direct sunshine using thin white fabric that still allows plenty of light through. If you are using grow lights, you may want to turn them down or back them off a little when starting a new culture. Once the culture is dense, they will generally want as much light as possible.

Making the Growth Medium

Making the medium is no more complicated than mixing the right water (see the "Using the Right Water" section below) with the right proportion of ingredients (if you're making your own medium from the recipes in AppendixA, the iron requires a little extra attention). If you're using pre-mixed nutrient mixes, it is truly simple.

Starting Your Tank

Get enough good water to fill your container about ¼ full.[14] For a 10-gallon tank and a 1-liter starter bottle, 10 liters is a good amount to start with. If you have pre-mixed Starter Mix, add 1.5 tablespoons of powder to every liter of water. For 10 liters, this means 15 tablespoons (that's one cup minus one tablespoon) of the Starter Mix in 10 liters of water. If you are using the pre-mixed Iron Juice, or if you make your own iron juice using citric acid, put two squeezes into your 10 liters and you're done. **This ratio – 7 1/2 tablespoons of starter powder and 1 squeeze of iron solution per 5 liters of water – is what to use whenever starting or expanding a culture.**

Note that if you are making your own nutrient mixes, it is best to measure out each ingredient separately, and use it right away. If you try to make a large amount of mix, and then scoop from that, the powders will tend to separate, and the proportions won't be right. The only way to prevent this is to blend and break down the powder to a uniform consistency. This can be done in a "dry" blender (the kind used to make flour); most kitchen blenders cannot do this!

---

14 Once you understand the growing-up process, you may decide to start with more or less than this. Expanding the culture in smaller steps means that the original algae medium is diluted less. Since this is the medium that the algae are adapted to, less dilution can reduce the shock to the algae if there is a big difference between the old and new media. Since the medium of the liter culture bottles sold by AlgaeLab.org is the same medium you will be using, larger dilutions are generally OK. The dilution suggested here (a half liter into 10 liters, i.e. 1:20) has been quite successful, but going to larger volumes faster may help avoid temperature swings by increasing the culture's mass, and should work as well.

Using the Right Water:

Using the wrong water will kill your Spirulina! The best source for the nutrient mixes we use is tap water, filtered through a filter medium such as activated carbon or ceramic (i.e. a Brita, Pur, Berkey, or other common water filtration systems). The only thing the filter has to do is remove the chlorination (this can also be done with dechlorination tablets, see below). Unchlorinated well or spring water should work as well, though you should still filter it if possible.

If you want to use unfiltered, chlorinated water, or low-mineral water sources such as distilled water, water filtered by reverse osmosis, or rain water, follow the instructions below. Some places have extremely "soft" water, which can have such low mineral content that it must also be treated as low-mineral water.

Of course, the water you use must be safe to drink!

To use chlorinated water: If you do not have a water filter, and the water source you have is chlorinated (e.g. tap water), you can dechlorinate the water as you would for an aquarium; any pet store will sell dechlorination kits that work well. (More advanced: The active ingredient is sodium thiosulfate; if you happen to have the pure crystalline stuff, use 0.1 to 0.3 grams per 10 liters of water to remove the chlorine.) If your water is chlorinated only with hypochlorite, and not chloramine (call your municipal water department), you can dechlorinate simply by letting the water sit at room temperature for 24 hours (bubbling or otherwise mixing if possible) to allow the chlorine to evaporate; it takes about a week to do the same if chloramine is present.

To use low-mineral water: If you want to use distilled water, rain water, or water that has been filtered using reverse osmosis, or if you live in a place with extremely "soft" water, you will need to add some extra minerals into the water to make up for what is missing from your water. This would be 0.1 g/L magnesium sulfate, 0.5 g/L potassium sulfate, and/or 0.1 g/L calcium chloride (or lime or plaster); the first two may not be necessary if the water is merely "soft". See Appendix A for more details.

Final note regarding "alkalized" water: Do not use "alkalized" water (e.g. from "Kangen" filters, etc.) – the pH is totally wrong for the Spirulina. If you don't know what this is, don't worry about it.

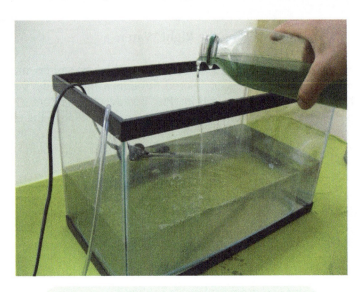

Figure 5: Fill your tank one-quarter full of medium and add half a liter of starter culture.

Angle the heater so that its top comes out of the water (if it is not "fully submersible", anything above the max level mark must be dry for your safety), where it can be more easily adjusted and read. **Plug in the bubbler. Mark the level of the water** on the side of the tank with an erasable marker.

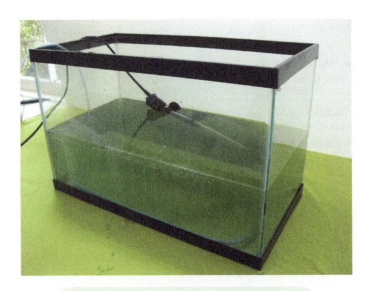

Figure 6: Add a cover and you're ready to grow!

It is usually a good idea to only pour in half of your bottle of starter (approximately half a liter), keeping the second half in reserve in case something goes wrong. It will grow up faster, though, if you use the whole bottle...

Finally, cover your tank. This should be fairly air-tight, with small holes to allow the bubbling air to escape. If it is installed correctly, the rush of air from these holes when the bubbling is on should be easily felt with the back of the hand. For an aquarium tank like the one pictured, a good approach is a piece of clear plexiglass, with small cut-outs for the heater cord & air tubing. Keep the cover on whenever possible, and keep the bubbling on at all times. This will help keep out potential invading algae and other micro-organisms, dust, bugs, etc.

Congratulation, your little guys are ready to grow!

A Few Things to Watch at the Start:

Temperature swings are most likely when the tank is only partially full, and before you've gotten used to how your heater works. Temperatures above 102F (39C) will kill your algae in a few hours. Using the thermometer, watch the temperature closely over the next few days, especially around noon on sunny days, when the sun can heat your tank up dramatically. This is something to keep in mind also in springtime and early summer, when solar heating can increase past the crucial 102F threshold. This is the time of year when we often get emails from sad algae farmers whose cultures have cooked! During the day, you will get best growth between 85-97F (29-36C). Use a heater if sunshine doesn't warm it up into this range. Generally, you will get higher growth at the higher end (around 97F), however, this is also potentially risky if the sun heats the culture above this temperature... Lower temperatures are better at night, which is the reason to use a timer to control the heater; temperatures below about 50F (10C), though, will harm the algae. If such low temperatures are a risk, either turn the heater down to 60F (16C) at night and leave it on, or put in a second heater in (this can be a smaller one, say 50W for a 10-gallon tank), set it to 60F, and leave it plugged in (i.e. do not use a timer). Low temperatures between 60-84F (16-29C) will not harm the algae, but will tend to slow their growth; this can be desirable if you want to "park" your culture for a while...

Keep an eye on the water level. If it drops significantly, add in fresh water (no nutrient mix!) to make up for evaporation, keeping the water level constant. If you cover the tank, you shouldn't have to do this more than once a week.

Be patient! Your culture will start out pretty dilute and pale green (see picture above), and gradually get denser and darker green. This stage can take a few weeks. If you check the pH at this stage (optional), it will start at around 8.5 and slowly rise as the days go by.

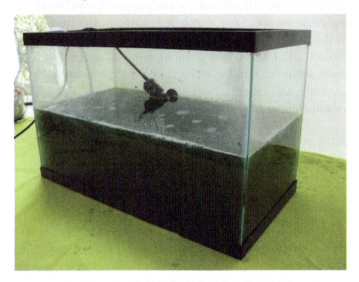

Figure 7: A dense culture: ready to be doubled in volume with fresh medium.

Growing Up the Culture

When the culture density gets high — to the level of the original AlgaeLab culture bottle, or less than 4 cm visibility (see the section on Measuring Algae Density below), or if it looks similar to the picture above — it's time to expand it. Add enough fresh medium to double the volume of the culture – for the first doubling of a 10-gallon tank, this amounts to 10 liters of water, 15 tablespoons of starter mix, and 2 squeezes of iron solution. For containers of other sizes, just use the proportions of 7 1/2 tablespoons of starter powder and 1 squeeze of iron solution per 5 liters of water, until you have doubled the volume.

If it is non-submersible, adjust the heater position to keep its top above water! Re-mark the water level so you can keep it constant by adding fresh water as before, to compensate for evaporation.

Wait until the culture is dense again, before doubling again. Keep going until the tank is full. If you want to more than double the culture — say you are going on a trip and won't be around for the next doubling time — that will generally work as well, it will just take longer for it to reach high density again...

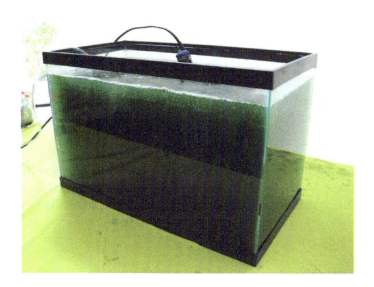

Figure 8: A full, dense culture: Always check the pH before harvesting!

Section 4: Harvesting Your Spirulina

Pre-Harvest SAFETY CHECKS

It is vitally important to carry out these safety checks prior to harvest! It is not safe to eat Spirulina if it is contaminated with other forms of algae, which may produce toxins.

This can generally be prevented by using a well-sealed tank cover (with only a few small air-release holes), **by using the exact medium recipe shown in Appendix A, and by verifiying that the pH of the culture is at least 10 before harvesting**. In my experience, a good tank cover, proper medium, and high pH quite reliably keeps dangerous species from growing in your tank.

However, **I strongly recommend getting a microscope to directly examine your culture**; in this way you can monitor the health of your culture (by counting the number of spirals in each strand, the more the better), and watch for any foreign algae. See Figure 9 for images of healthy Spirulina, obtained using inexpensive microscopes; see the below section for recommendations regarding microscopes for Spirulina cultivation. Be on the lookout for anything that is green but not shaped like Spirulina. You may also see fragments of Spirulina spirals; a few of these are OK, but if they are increasing in number, it may be an indication that something in your system (pumps, splashing, etc.) may be breaking up the spirals, which is not good -- see "Shear and Strand Breakage" in Section 8 for more details. Some types of potentially harmful algae have round cells about as big across as as Spirulina spirals are wide, so at 100x they are little more than green dots; at 400x they can be examined much more closely (though they are still small).

Microscopes for Checking Spirulina Culture:

There are many types of microscopes available, some more appropriate for looking at your culture than others. The most important consideration is magnification; what you need is at least 100x, but 400x is much better. Magnification is equal to the eyepice magnification multiplied by the objective magnification. In inexpensive microscopes suitable for Spirulina, there is typically one eyepiece with a magnification of 10x, and several objectives with magnifications ranging from 4x to 40x, resulting in a total magnification from 40x to 400x. The smaller magnification objectives are useful for seeing a larger area of the culture, to find objects of interest that can be zoomed in on with the higher-power objectives.

FYI: Some microscope companies make extravagant claims about magnfication in scopes with digital video outputs, confusing the size that images can be projected onto computer monitors with true optical magnification. The actual magnification of eyepieces and objectives is what counts!

The next consideration is whether to spend a little more to get an "inverted" microscope. In an inverted microscope, the objective lens "looks up" through the microscope slide; in a normal microscope, the objectives look down onto the sample. Because the curved upper surface of a water droplet forms a wobbly extra lens, if you want to look down into a water droplet you must use a cover slide (a wafer-thin piece of glass) on top of it. This takes some care, and it is why inverted 'scopes are a big improvement -- not only can you just put a droplet on a slide and look at it immediately, but you can put multiple droplets (if you have multiple cultures) on one slide and quickly survey many cultures.

Another signficant upgrade is to get a mechanical stage, which allows you to controllably scan your view across the sample. Also, many new microscopes have digital cameras built in, and many can plug into your computer; it is also possible to add a digital camera later, though, and you may be able to get usable images just by pointing your digital camera down the eyepiece!

At the time of this writing, a basic 400x microscope can be had for $80; a stage and digital camera can be added for a little more. A 400x inverted scope (without stage or camera) can be had for $200.

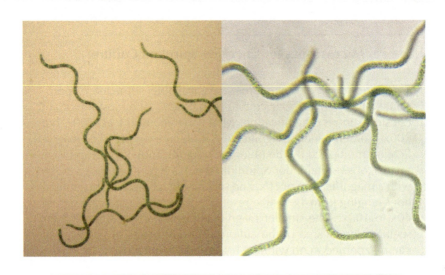

Figure 9: Healthy Spirulina spirals in the microscope: on the left, at 100x magnification; on the right, 400x magnification. At the higher magnification, note that you can see individual cells in the filaments.

I have looked at many sorts of algae cultures under the microscope, and constantly examine our Spirulina cultures. At the time of this writing, in Spirulina cultures grown in the medium described in this book, I have only seen non-Spiurlina organisms (other types of algae) in a few cases where the pH was below 10.

Check the pH (see the following section on pH for details); if it is below 10, don't harvest yet. pH will start at around 8.5 for fresh medium, then rise fairly quickly over the next few weeks, hitting 10 in a month or so. pH should continue to rise after that, but only very slowly, after reaching 10+. If it is 11 or above (which won't happen for several months or more after the first grow-up), you will get better growth if you replace the medium (see below). See the "pH, and How To Check It" section below for how to check pH.

pH, and How To Check It:

pH represents the balance between acidity and basicity in water. The lower the pH, the more acidic the water; the higher, the more basic. A value of 7 means neutral — a balance between acid and base. Many biochemical reactions depend critically on pH, so all organisms have a limited pH range in which they can live. Spirulina is specially adapted to grow in extremely high pH — 11 or even higher. Very few organisms can grow at a pH of 10+, so maintaining your culture at 10+ pH helps keep your culture clear of potentially harful critters.

How to measure pH? There are two basic options: pH strips, and pH meters. For beginners, and the economically-minded, pH test strips are a good option, and they are easy to use. However, the most commonly-available wide pH strips cover a wide range of pH values (typically, 1-14), and don't distinguish well between the critical pH values around 10. For this reason it is best to use short-range pH strips for Spirulina growth; pHydrion sells strips that distinguishes the pH range 9.2-10.6 (microessentiallab.com), and can handily tell you if your culture is in the "safe" range. These are the type provided in the AlgaeLab kits.

The more "pro" option is to use a pH meter; these can cost anywhere from $30 to $2000 or more. The more expensive ones are more accurate, but for general purposes the cheaper types are fine. All pH meters require fairly frequent re-calbration, so be sure to buy "buffers" — solutions of compounds that maintain a fairly accurate pH even if somewhat contaminated — at 4, 7, and 10 pH. Keep the probe tip submerged in the 4 pH solution when you are not using it; rinse it off well between uses, and don't let the probe tip (the "bulb" part, usually made of glass) dry out. If it does dry out, or get contaminated with any sort of sticky stuff, you'll need to re-condition it, with a soak in pH 4 buffer, or in reconditioning solution if necessary.

Harvest Basics

When the tank is full, density is high, and pH is 10+, you are ready to harvest! There are many ways to harvest the algae. The basic idea is simply to pass the culture through a fine filter, catching the Spirulina spirals and returning the filtered water to the culture. Some extra nutrients (Make-Up Mix, see Appendix A for recipe) are added back to the culture, in proportion to the amount taken out, to make up for those lost in the harvested Spirulina. The harvested Spirulina then gets a final squeeze to push out any remaining water, and is ready to eat!

This means that a harvesting set-up requires five things:

1. A way of getting the water out of the tank and to the filter.

Getting the culture out of the tank can be done using a siphon (see below), or a simple aquarium pump (these can cost $10 or less). If you want to pump over a vertical rise of a foot or more, you may want to consider using a diaphragm pump of the type used to pump out boat bilges; these are highly effective and cost $80 or less. You'll need to be able to control the rate at which the culture is pumped so that the filter won't overflow.

2. An effective filter.

All that is required for catching the Spirulina spirals is a filter with openings 50 microns across or less. Although cheese cloth or coffee filters will work to some extent, they are difficult to clean, and much of the precious blue-green stuff will end up stuck in the material. The most convenient and inexpensive solution is to use nylon screen printing fabric, with a fineness of 300 mesh, also known as 120 thread. This type of cloth is easy to clean and can be used hundreds of times. It can be sewn into the shape of a cone or sock to speed and/or simplify the process, but a 1'x1' square of the cloth will work as well, as shown below.

3. A way of getting the filtered culture back into the tank.

This can be as simple as dumping a bucket back into the tank, or simply doing the filtration over the tank so that the filtered culture simply falls back into the tank.

4. Nutrients to make up for those in the harvested spirulina.

As your Spirulina spirals grow, they absorb nutrients from the medium; after you harvest, it is necessary to add new nutrients to the medium to make up for those in the harvested algae. This is how the optimal growth medium can be maintained through multiple harvests. Buy Make-Up Mix powder from AlgaeLab.org, or see the recipe in Appendix A to make your own.

5. A way to squeeze out the remaining water.

If you are using a simple harvest cloth, this is very simple to do; just be sure to design any support for the harvest cloth so that it allows for some squeezing of the harvested stuff when you're done filtering. This is easily done if the harvest cloth is removable from any support. As shown below, support for the harvest cloth is not necessary, although many growers have used a large sieve to support the cloth, which eliminates the need for the clips.

Harvesting, Step by Step

Here we will describe probably the simplest way that meets all these requirements, step by step, so that you'll understand exactly what is required; then we'll talk about variants that may speed things up or enable bigger harvests.

For this approach you'll need:

- A bucket holding 2.5 or 5 gallons,
- Approximately 18" of 3/4" tubing (preferably clear),
- A 1'x1' square of screen printing fabric, 300 mesh (120 thread) or close,
- 4 clothespins

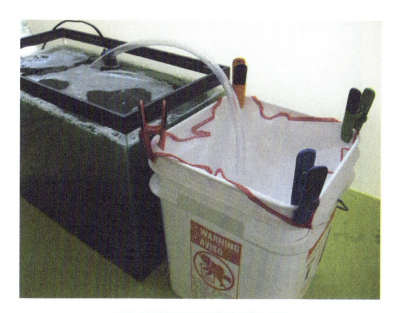

Figure 10: Set up for harvest.

Set up the bucket next to the tank. Wash your hands and wrists thoroughly. Use a sieve to eliminate any clumps or lumps from the tank before harvesting. The process goes faster (and you can harvest more Spirulina) if the bucket can be placed lower than the tank; 2"-6" works well. If the bucket is at just the right level, the siphon will run as fast as it can without overflowing the filter, and the bucket won't overflow; this way you can just get the siphon going, and come back to it when it's done. In the beginning, though, and any time you want your Spirulina as fast as possible, you'll want to have the bucket low, and you'll control the flow rate, either with your thumb on the tube end, or by raising and lowering the tube end. Use clips to secure the harvest filter cloth across the open top of the bucket, allowing it to droop down by 3 inches or more as seen above. You can also use a large sieve to hold and support the harvest cloth.

If there are a lot of clumps in the culture, you may want to filter these out above the filter cloth; just use a strainer or screen; the splash screens used to keep frying oil from splashing out of a pan can work well for this purpose, when placed above the harvest cloth.

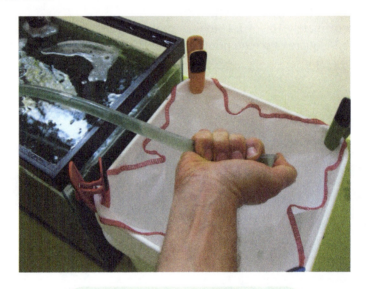

Figure 11: Siphon ready to go...

Use a 3/4" diameter tube as a siphon, by immersing it in the culture and allowing it to fill *completely* with culture; this will happen if the tube is in a U shape, with both ends facing up; it won't work if there's a loop in the tube. Once the tube is full, plug one end of it with your thumb, then pull that end out while keeping the other end immersed. Keeping it plugged, place the tube end into the lowest part of the filter cloth and let go. If this end of the tube is below the culture level, this should form a siphon, which will draw the culture into the filter. You can also use a small pump in place of the siphon, if it's more convenient.

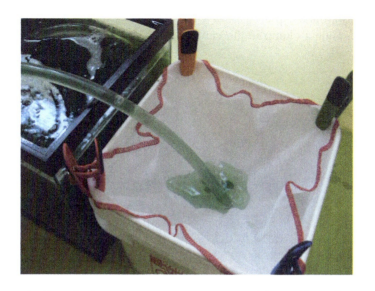

Figure 12: Siphon starting to flow; note flecks of green, these are Spirulina spirals collecting on the filter cloth!

Don't let the filtered medium fill up to the point that it touches the bottom of the filter cloth! Keep an eye on it, and stop the flow before that happens.

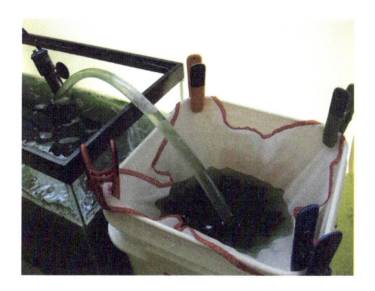

Figure 13: Level between tank and liquid in harvest cloth has equalized, so flow has paused...

Gather the spirulina captured in the cloth together by raising the edges and gently shaking, forming a clump in the center. You can use a spoon to scrape it all together instead.

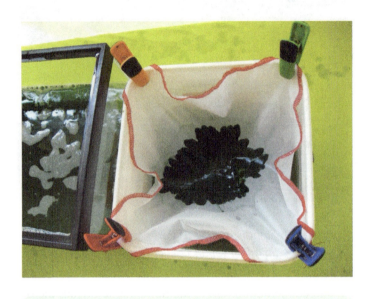

Figure 14: Remaining medium has drained out, leaving still-wet Spirulina, ready to be squeezed...

Using a motion as if milking an udder, gently squeeze the slurry into a ball in the center, and give this ball a firm squeeze to release most of the remaining medium. Stop when you see green liquid coming through. If you squeeze too much, broken Spirulina strands will be forced through the openings of the cloth; if you squeeze too little, the harvested paste may have a slightly bitter taste due to the baking soda in the medium. You will soon learn the correct amount of pressure to use.

Open the cloth. There it is – fresh Spirulina that you grew! If the Spirulina sticks to itself better than the cloth, and easily forms a compact mass, this means that the Spirulina spirals are nice and long, which indicates that they are doing well – not being starved for nutrients or otherwise stressed (which can make them brittle), or being broken up by shear (caused by pumps or violent splashing/bubbling).

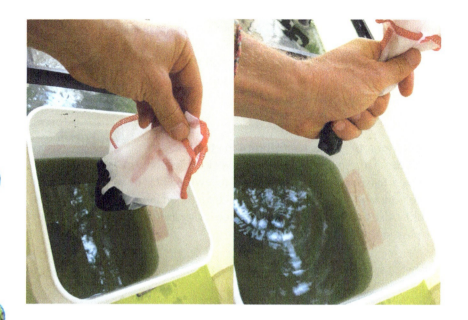

Figure 15: Gathering up the Spirulina spirals into the center of the filter cloth, squeezing out the remaining liquid.

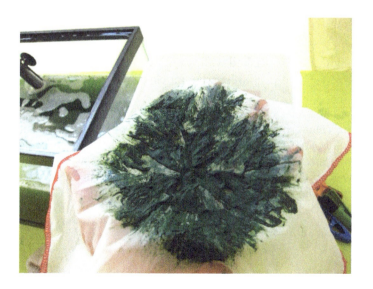

Figure 16: Fresh Spirulina.

If you desire a larger harvest, repeat these steps, or build a larger harvest setup (see suggestions below...). If you want to be able to harvest again soon, though, **don't pass more than half the tank volume through the filter cloth at one time**, or the remaining culture may become too thin to grow back quickly. On the other hand, if you plan to wait longer than usual before the next harvest, thinning the culture is a good idea...

Use a tablespoon to gather all the Spirulina together and scoop it up. Assess the volume of the harvested spirulina. **For every tablespoon of fresh spirulina harvested, mix 1 teaspoon of the "Make-Up" mix with a liter or so of water and pour it into the tank** (alternately, mix it with the culture medium that passed through the filter cloth). **Also add a squeeze of iron juice for every five liters (1 1/3 gallons) of culture passed through the filter.**

The harvested spirulina should be dark blue-green. If it is not, do not eat it.

Enjoy the spirulina! Put it in your smoothie, mix it in soup or sauces after cooking – avoid exposure to high temperatures to maintain the nutrient content. See the Spirulina Recipes section for preparation ideas. Keep in mind that **fresh spirulina is like raw eggs or raw meat, and spoils very quickly**; do not touch it unless your hands are very clean, and refrigerate immediately if you're not going to eat it right away. It will last in the fridge (bottom shelf, less than 40F) for up to a week. If frozen, it lasts indefinitely; if dehydrated (and kept dry), it will last for about a year, longer if kept in an airtight container. It's not hard to tell if it does go bad – it smells like rotten eggs.

The harvest cloth can be washed with warm water and a bit of soap, or it can be placed in the top rack of your dishwasher for cleaning.

Some Spirulina growers "clean" their harvested algae before eating it, to rinse off any remaining culture medium before eating it. If you intend to do this, do not squeeze the Spirulina, but instead immerse the freshly harvested stuff in a container of clean fresh water, mix it up well (but not violently, as this could break the strands), to wash off the Spirulina strands, then use above harvest technique again, to extract the Spirulina from the rinse water. After such a rinse, the squeezing step is optional.

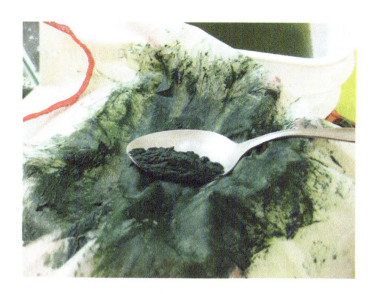

Figure 17: Ready to eat!

Section 5: Culture Maintenance

Basic Maintenance

Keeping your culture happy doesn't take much work, but it's important to keep an eye on it, as shifts can happen unexpectedly – if, say, a few warm sunny days, or a few cold, cloudy days in a row cause the temperature to swing dangerously, or if the bubbler gets unplugged – and sometimes quick action is required.

In general, though, these are the main things to keep track of:

- **Keep a healthy back-up culture of a liter or so in a bright but not directly sun-lit place.** Maintain it as you would newly-arrived culture (see Section 3). Swap it out for fresh healthy culture every few weeks or so. If If you have two or more tanks, or a friend who also grows, you may be able to get away without this.

- **Add more fresh water (without added nutrients) occasionally to replace evaporated water** and keep the level of the culture constant.

- As your Spirulina grows, some will stick to the walls, bubbler, heater, etc., and floating clumps can form. The algae often produce transparent jelly-like polysaccharides, which also tend to stick to things or form floating masses. This is normal, though they can form more of this stuff if they are stressed, or if you let a thick culture sit without harvesting for a while. **These floating clumps can be scooped up with a strainer** to separate them from the culture for disposal. If there are many, use the siphon to draw larger quantities of medium through a screen to capture the clumps, or clean out the tank. **If more clumps than usual are forming, check the pH, and think about what might be amiss with the growing conditions (insufficient mixing, enough/too much light, incorrect nutrients, high/low temperatures, etc.).** If this problem persists, renew the culture medium as described below. Put the clumps in your compost.

- If excess clumps of spirulina can be seen at the bottom, or if there is too much crud accumulating in general, **the whole culture can be siphoned temporarily into buckets or other (clean!) containers while the tank inside is cleaned**. I recommend thoroughly cleaning the tank every month.

- **When you remove Spirulina clumps, add in "Make-Up" mix in proportion to the spirulina removed in this way** – 1 tsp powder, and a squeeze of iron juice, per two tablespoons of algae gunk removed. Clumps that aren't blue-green don't count. Mix it in some water before adding it to the tank.

- White, chalky limescale deposits often develop on the heater over time. These can be removed by soaking in a 10% vinegar solution, or by using a vinegar-soaked sponge.

Harvesting regularly (half the tank every 2-3 days) is the best way to keep a clean, nice-looking culture. When Spirulina cells split they have a natural electric charge on them that prevents strands from clumping together, which is slowly overcome by accumulated molecular junk on their outside surfaces if they don't split again soon. They also tend to produce more jelly when they get excessively dense. If you harvest regularly, the Spirulina will keep growing and splitting all the time, and will produce less jelly.

Renewing the Culture Medium

If the pH of the culture is 11 or above, or if you have any reason to think that the medium chemistry is off (i.e. the culture is yellowish or thin, and doesn't grow well), you will need to replace the medium. This is no more difficult than harvesting...

Mix up enough medium to fill approximately half of your growth container. For a ten-gallon tank, this means combining 30 tablespoons of starter mix, 4 squeezes of iron juice, and 20 liters of filtered water. Move the heater in to the new medium to start equalizing the temperature. **Run the entire culture through the harvest cloth**; since your tank is probably bigger than your bucket, you'll have to do this in stages. If there are a lot of clumps (the usual scenario), use a strainer or screen to remove them from the culture; this can be done prior to filtering, or one of the round flat screens used to keep frying oil from splashing out of a pan can be used for this purpose.

After each stage of filtering, put the cloth with the harvested Spirulina immediately into the new medium — do not squeeze it — and swish it around to release the cells into the water. Pour the old medium into your compost pile. If there are a lot of clumps at the bottom, you may want to sacrifice that part of the culture, as clumps and polysaccharide jelly tend to encourage more clumping...

Putting it in Park: Resting Your Culture

Unlike most pets, you generally don't need a sitter for your Spirulina (also, most pets won't feed *you*...). **If you won't be able to tend to your Spirulina for a while (more than a week), you can put your culture into "stasis" mode**, and it should be fine for a few weeks, or even months. The main idea is to thin out the culture, and slow down its rate of growth so it won't use up all its nutrients and starve. The rate of growth is slowed by reducing the temperature of the culture, and the amount of light it receives.

To do this, give it a good harvest to reduce its density (take it down to 5+ cm density if you're measuring), and turn off the high-temperature (timed) heater. If you're using a low-temperature heater to protect from low temperatures, leave that one on. Use some thin white fabric to protect the culture from direct sunshine, but allowing some light through. As long as the culture doesn't experience any extreme temperatures – less than 50F (7C) or more than 102F (39C) – it should be fine for quite a while; temperatures around 65-80F (18-27C) are best for keeping your algae alive while minimizing their growth rate. Make sure, though, you have a healthy reserve culture bottle in a safe place, just in case...

Section 6: Alternative Harvest Techniques

The harvest technique described above is the most basic possible, using the minimum of equipment. You can probably come up with improvements using a little more gear. Here are some possibilities:

1. Putting a spigot on the bottom of the tank. This makes the siphon unnecessary, and allows you to completely drain the tank before you move it. This is difficult to do in an aquarium tank, but other designs (e.g. iced tea dispensers) make it possible. Beware, though, that even a short length of pipe leading out of the tank can create a "dead zone" that has no circulation – this will be a place where all sorts of crud will tend to accumulate, so you'll have to clean it frequently!

2. Using a pump instead of a siphon. This can be done by suspending a harvest cloth over the top of your culture, and then pumping the culture up and through the cloth using a cheap aquarium pump (less than $10). This type of pump can damage Spirulina spirals (see "Shear and Strand Breakage", p.51) if they pass through it many times, but it's OK for harvesting, which is a one-way trip... Just turn on the pump and let it run for a while! Just be careful not to leave it running too long and harvest too much, as that can slow re-growth and delay the next harvest.

3. Improving the shape of the harvest cloth. The screen printing fabric can be sewn like any other fabric. Make it into a cone or sock (cylindrical) shape – which one depends on your particular harvesting setup – to speed up harvesting by allowing you to create a greater depth of culture inside the cloth, and increasing the surface area through which the culture can flow.

4. Drying the Spirulina. If you want to preserve Spirulina for a long time without freezing it, you'll need to dry it. The best way to do this is to put the Spirulina paste into a spaghetti maker and squeeze out long strings onto drying pans; put these in a dehydrator, or an oven at the lowest temperature setting to dry. If the weather is hot and sunny, you can sun-dry as well. Make sure that the Spirulina are thoroughly dried in less than three hours, and then store them immediately in air-tight containers; they will go bad quickly if damp, especially at high temperature! If stored in this way, Spirulina should keep for 2-3 years or more.

A note about the timing of your harvest: Spirulina, like all algae, tend to accumulate energy-storage products (carbohydrates and oils) during the course of the day as they soak in light energy, and then use this energy to grow and/or split at night. For this reason, they have the highest protein levels at dawn, and the lowest at dusk. The changes are not huge, though (about 25%), and you may want the oils (which are rich in healthy omega-3 fatty acids). So you can harvest early for more protein, later for more oil, or not worry about it...

Section 7: Expanding Your Set-Up

General Considerations for Expansion

Once you have one tank going, naturally your appetite for fresh Spirulina, and the appetite of those around you, will start to soar – time to expand your setup! The easy way is to just put more tank in your windows – see Figure 1. There are many possible containers for algae you might want to consider, though. Other than the obvious considerations of dimensions, cost, and aesthetics, here are three things to keep in mind regarding your growth container:

Light path – How far does light have to go to reach every part of your culture? If this is more than 6", you'll have trouble getting your culture very dense, as much of your culture will be in the dark once the algae start to grow. If light comes into your culture from both sides, then 12" is the maximum thickness we recommend; the tank can be taller and wider, though. If your tank has a shorter light path (see Figure 18), the culture will be able to get proportionately denser.

Cleaning – Sometimes we see very inventive designs involving long lengths of narrow tubing, or labyrinths of channels sealed into plastic sheets, and we wonder how the designers intend to remove accumulated crud and algae stuck to the walls. Inevitably, you will need to scrub it out occasionally (monthly is best), so take this into account in your design!

Material Compatibility with Algae, and Food – Many building materials include additives intended to keep microorganisms (especially fungus) from growing on them; these additives can kill your algae as well. Examples are almost every kind of silicone sealant you can find in the hardware store – use aquarium-grade, or food-grade silicone only! – and some types of non-food-grade tubing. In general, use food-grade materials wherever possible, aquarium-grade materials at minimum. Materials rated for contact with potable water are generally OK. Research any material you use to make sure it is safe for long-term contact with food. We like glass aqaurium tanks because they usually use only glass (which is generally safe if not coated), and pure, aquarium-grade silicone.

Also, **even small amounts of copper, silver, or zinc in the medium** – for example, even a small piece of copper pipe, or the use of water stored in a copper vessel – **will kill your algae,** so avoid those materials. This includes bronze, a common material for valves, spigots, etc., which is rich in copper and zinc. Galvanized metal, which is covered in zinc, should also be avoided.

You may wish to avoid plastics with extractable compounds such as BPA as well – research this on your own if you don't know what I'm talking about, it's a controversial topic.

Ideas for Growth Containers

You probably have a few ideas for Spirulina growth containers already; a scan of the internet (and the U.S. patent office) will turn up a fantastical array of algae growth system concepts — check them out!

The following pages present a run-down of a few common (and/or cool) approaches, with their pros and cons...

Glass Aquariums

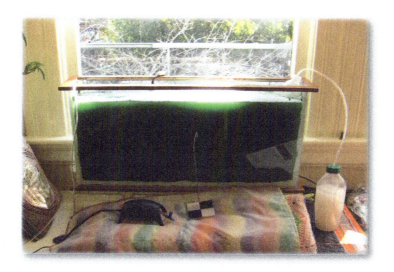

Figure 18: Custom-made glass aquarium with relatively short (4", 10 cm) light path.

Advantages:
- Small aquariums are very cheap (about $15 for a 10-gallon tank) and easy to obtain; you may have one lying around...
- Materials of commercial aquariums – glass and aquarium-grade silicone sealant – are likely to be compatible with algae growth, and your health.
- It's not difficult to make your own glass aquarium, with a shorter light path (see above) for denser growth...

Disadvantages:
- Larger tanks are much more expensive, so you may want to consider other approaches when scaling up.
- Larger tanks are usually more than 12" wide, so their light path is too long, unless you put lights inside the tank...
- If you build your own tanks, be sure to use aquarium- or food-grade sealant!
- Glass tanks are difficult to ship.

Plastic Bottles

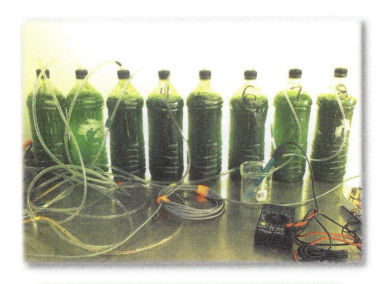

Figure 19: A test of eight different growth media, using identical soda bottles. They are arrayed in front of a horizontal fluorescent light fixture.

Advantages:
- Cheap and usually lying around.
- Fit nicely on a window sill.
- Easily mixed with aquarium-style bubbling system; one air pump can bubble a dozen or more.
- Perfect for keeping your reserve culture, especially as they have lids – just drill a hole for the air tube, another for the air output tube, and you have a well-isolated container relatively safe from contamination.[15]
- Good for growth experiments – try different media, temperatures, etc.

Disadvantages:
- Small. It's a lot of work to harvest/clean large numbers of bottles.
- Not easy to wash out thoroughly - get a bottle brush!

---

15   To make it totally safe from contamination, though, you have to put the bubbling air through a sterilizing filter.

Hanging Plastic Bags

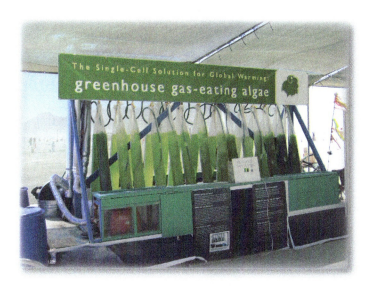

Figure 20: Chlorophyll Collective exhibit, Burning Man Art Festival, 2007. Scenedesmus algae, absorbing pollutants from generator exhaust.

Advantages:
- *Cheap and easy to obtain and make — 12" wide polyethylene mailing tubes cost less than $1 for 6'+!*
- *Can be fairly tall ~6', so volume can be appreciable.*
- *Short light path.*
- *Bubbling is effective for mixing and gas exchange.*
- *Heat seals can be angled to make a cone bottom; if you bubble at the bottom of the cone, settling can be greatly reduced.*
- *Can also be laid on their sides for a horizontal photobioreactor...*

Disadvantages:
- *Must build strong structure to hang bags.*
- *For multi-month lifetime, must use UV-stabilized greenhouse film ("four season") instead of tubes, but need a heat sealer to make bags.*
- *Doesn't scale well: large volumes requires many tubes.*

Free-Standing Vertical Tube(s)

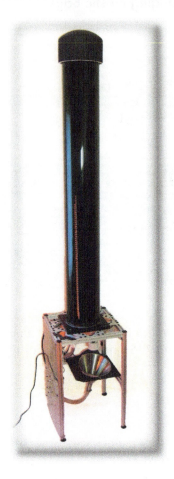

Figure 21: Prototype of an AlgaeLab/Spiralife project to develop a personal Spirulina photobioreactor system.

Advantages:
- Can be fairly tall: 6'+, so volume can be appreciable.
- Short light path.
- Attractive look.
- Long-lasting, if material is UV-stabilized, or kept out of sun.
- Bubbling is effective for mixing and gas exchange.

Disadvantages:
- Hard plastic tubes are expensive.
- Doesn't scale well: large volumes requires many tubes.
- Overheating may be an issue in intense sunlight.
- If sun-exposed, must use UV-stabilized plastic.

Open Ponds

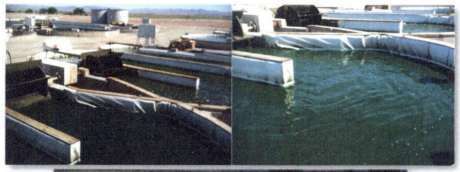

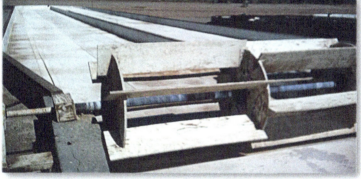

Figure 22: Some examples of open commercial prodiction ponds, of various sizes, including the paddlewheels. All commercial Spirulina farms use these types of ponds.

Advantages:
- Least expensive approach for large-scale production.
- Easily scaled to very large facilities (1-3+ acres per pond).
- Can be covered by greenhouse for better control of temperature, evaporation, and contamination.
- Evaporation from pond surface helps cool the pond on hot days.

Disadvantages:
- Much greater potential for contamination due to blown dust, birds, insects, etc. – close monitoring required.
- More evaporation.
- Shallow depth requires special carbonation system.
- Significant construction project.

Alternative Mixing Techniques

You don't necessarily have to use bubbles for mixing. There are a lot of ways to stir up your culture and keep your spirals floating freely. The simplest Spirulina farms don't even need electricity; at the Simplicity Spirulina Farm in Auroville, India local women stir the culture with special brooms three times a day, with no other mixing! You can do something similar, but if you want maximum growth, or have a day job, you'll want some automatic form of mixing.

There are three basic ways to do this: bubbles, pumps, or propellers/paddles. Each has advantages and disadvantages.

Mixing with bubbles is a particularly easy way to mix a culture using off-the-shelf aquarium gear, which is why we use it in our kits and recommend it for small-scale installations in general. One great advantage of bubbling is that it helps the algae to breathe. Algae breathe in carbon dioxide and breathe out oxygen, so it is important to deliver the former into the culture, and the latter out. (See the Carbon Dioxide section below for details.) This gas exchange happens through air-water surfaces; by providing more air-water contact area, bubbles accelerate this process. Another great thing about bubbling systems is their flexibility; you can move bubblers around easily, and put more in any place which doesn't seem to be getting enough mixing. The main consideration is to make sure that every part of the culture volume is moving approximately equally. **It is best to avoid having dead-end pipes or other small semi-enclosed spaces within your culture**, where crud will tend to accumulate; this crud can eventually cause problems in your culture if it begins to decay. This also applies to where you put the bubblers; make sure that the bubbles are as widely distributed on the bottom of the tank as possible, and if possible make the turbulence greatest on walls and other surfaces where algae might otherwise tend to stick. Bubbling works best, and is most efficient (in terms of cost and energy usage) when the culture vessel is generally taller than it is wide. But bubbling can be considerably less energy-efficient than well-designed pumping or paddle/propeller systems, which is why it is not often used in large commercial systems.

Using a pump is potentially even easier than bubbling – just suck water from the bottom of the culture, or the end of a tube or channel, and feed it back to the top of the culture, or the beginning of your tube or channel. This can provide decent mixing (though, like bubbling, this depends strongly on the geometry), with one big caveat: most inexpensive pumps (which use centrifugal force to pump water) will chop your Spirulina spirals into little pieces quite quickly, ultimately killing your culture! If you wish to pump Spirulina culture, try "low-shear" type pumps, like a diaphragm pump, or a "positive displacement" pump. The former can be inexpensive and relatively easy to find in the form of bilge pumps for boats. Another potentially low-shear way to pump your Spirulina is to use rising bubbles inside a tube to lift the culture up; this is called an airlift pump. However, all of these pump types involve some shear. Don't take for granted the low-shear nature of any pump – test it out on some real culture and observe the culture under a microscope to see if it is getting shredded...

Using a propeller or paddle is also pretty simple. This is how the pros do it, using paddlewheels to push their culture around open racetrack-shaped ponds. They do this because it is the most energy-efficient way to mix, it can be extremely low shear, and it mixes the algae quite uniformly. By maintaining a relatively uniform speed everywhere in the racetrack pond, the algae are kept in suspension. For a small-scale approach, you can use kitchen mixers (designed to mount on pots and stir them so that the cook can do something else), or magnetic mixers as is often done in a lab (which, if done properly, can minimize any chance of contamination). Just watch the speed of the paddle or propeller tip – too fast and you'll shear the Spirulina spirals. A maximum speed of about 3 feet (1m) per second will be fine; above that, you'd better do some testing.

For more information about algae mixing, see our book for more advanced algae farmers...

Section 8: Spirulina Growing Tips

Here is all the useful additonal information I can think of that you might want to know, organized by topic.

Light

When your culture is growing well and fairly thick, it will grow best when exposed to maximum sunshine – the more the better. In fact, you will find that growth is roughly proportional to the number of hours the tank spends in direct sunshine. This is an important factor for choosing where to put the algae tank. A greenhouse is ideal, next best is a south-facing window that gets a lot of sun, without any trees, plants, or buildings that block the sun.

In some cases you can overdo it with light, though. A lot of direct sunshine (or other bright light) can hurt the algae when the culture is thin or the algae are otherwise stressed (e.g. immediately after putting your starter into your tank, or when pH is high, temperature is low, or nutrients are off). Also, a lot of sunshine can cause the tank temperature to climb too high (see below). If this starts happening, shade your algae a little (thin white fabric is best, to ensure that not too much light is lost), then give them sun again for maximum productivity, once the problem is fixed.

You can also use artificial illumination to grow your algae. Spirulina grows best with a lot of light, so be prepared to dump in a lot of wattage if you want rapid growth! Use high-efficiency light sources (fluorescent or LEDs) to avoid running up your electric bill. It is important to put the light source inside or as close to the culture as possible, both to maximize light absorption and to take advantage of the heat they generate. For example, one of our AlgaeLab growers got excellent growth using fluorescent bulbs inside re-purposed spaghetti jars immersed in the tank.

One of the main considerations (and something that I am often asked about) is what wavelengths/colors are best for growing Spirulina. Most land plants need both red and blue light to thrive, and chlorophyll absorbs both red and blue light. Blue-green algae, such as spirulina, have special accessory pigments called phycocyanins and allophycocyanins, which allow them to capture more red and orange light (and to a lesser extent yellow and green) than green plants. They do have chlorophyll (essentially the same as green plants' chlorophyll), so they can also use blue light.

Ordinary "grow lights", which are optimized for green land plants, are not particularly good for growing Spirulina or other blue-green algae (though they will work). A light with more red and orange light — i.e. a "warmer" color — will be more efficient for growth, as a higher fraction of the light will be absorbed. Another approach would be to use white light supplemented by a red-orange light source (peaking at 620-650 nm), to hit the phyco-pigments better, or red light (650-680 nm). Wavelengths longer than 680 nm are not useful for photosynthesis. I have had success with the "warmer" colored compact fluorescents, as well as red LEDs. I have also found that any whitish source of light will work, although efficiency can vary somewhat.

In general, though, the color of the light source is not as important in my experience as getting the nutrients and temperature right, and providing LOTS of light, which is easier using sunshine. Direct sunshine is about 100x brighter (~100,000 lux) than the light in what would be considered a bright artificially-lit room (1000 lux). It's hard to compete with the sun! Virtually every commercial algae grower uses sunlight for large-scale cultivation.

Temperature

Temperature is also very important. The AlgaeLab algae (*Arthrospira platensis* from the NCMA culture collection) seem to prefer temperatures around 92 Fahrenheit (33 Centigrade). It is often good to keep your temperature below that, though, as the temperature can rise quickly when the tank is struck by direct sun. Above about 102F (39C) they tend to clump up and turn yellowish, indicating stress; just a few degrees higher and they die quickly. If this happens, lower the temperature, strain out the clumps, add in nutrients as if you just harvested, protect them from large amounts of sun and from extreme temperatures, and they will bounce back and turn blue-green again. High temperatures, caused by unexpected increases in sun exposure, or malfunctioning heaters, is one of the most common ways in which home-grown Spirulina cultures have been lost so far. Keep in mind the extra heat the tank will receive when cloudy days become sunny, or when the angle of the sun changes to give the tank more hours of illumination.

Moderately low temperatures are not harmful – in fact, because they slow down the algae's metabolism, they can help keep them alive without feeding/mixing, if live spirulina need to be stored for a few days (or longer) – but they won't grow well. As a general rule, growth is slow below about 80F (27C). The algae should be protected from temperatures below about 50F (10C), however. If such low temperatures are expected, keep the culture at 55F (13C) or higher either by keeping the main heater on at night, set at the lower temperature, or by using a second heater set at that temperature, plugged it into the wall (don't use a timer), so that it can turn on whenever the temperature drops too low. The second option is generally better, unless you think you can remember to turn the heater up and down every morning and evening! Such a second heater can usually be considerably smaller than the main heater (we often use one half the size), unless the tank's environment is extremely cold.

It is also worth noting that sudden, drastic changes in temperature – such as putting live Spirulina into particularly cold medium when changing the medium – can wipe out your culture very quickly. Warm up medium that is particularly cold (<65F) before you transfer Spirulina into it, and avoid any sudden changes to the algae's environment.

Carbon Dioxide

Carbon dioxide (CO_2) is an essential nutrient for the growth of any plant, including Spirulina. Practically all commercial Spirulina growers bubble extra CO_2 into their cultures to accelerate growth; it is generally thought that the proper delivery of CO_2 into a culture can roughly double the growth rate. This is a major expense for the growers, though, and it adds significant complexity to their systems.

There is a considerable (constantly increasing...) amount of carbon dioxide in the atmosphere. If your culture is well mixed (i.e. if your bubbler is working properly), this is generally adequate for good growth. **If you have a very high-sunshine setup that is growing well, and you desire higher growth, you may want to experiment with carbon dioxide supplementation to increase the growth further.** You can use bottled CO_2 from a welding shop – use a very low-pressure regulator, as you'll need less than 1 psi (1 psi of pressure per 2 feet of depth is required), be careful to bubble it in slowly, and use it only in a well-ventilated area. Much cheaper, and safer, is to use the gas escaping from a fermentation process – brewing, yogurt-making, sour dough starter, whiskey mash, etc. Just take the output from the fermenter and feed the bubbles into the tank; you'll get much better absorption, though, if you trap the gas in contact with the culture; one way to do this is to float a membrane with weighted edges, or any dome-shaped object with its edges submerged, positioned where it catches the bubbles; in this way the CO_2-rich fermentation gas can be kept in contact with the culture much longer than if the bubbles simply rise and escape. Also, if you are supplementing with CO_2 you must keep an eye on the pH, as it will tend to drop, making the culture vulnerable to invasion by contaminating microorganisms if the pH falls below 10. This is especially true at night, when it is better to turn any CO_2 supplementation off, as algae only use it when they are photosynthesizing.

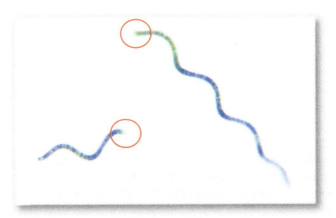

Figure 23: Examples of strand breakage, indicated by red circles. Note the neat, tapered unbroken ends in comparison. 400x.

Shear and Strand Breakage

Spirulina is made of lots of tiny cells (about 8 microns across) connected in filaments that form a spiral shape. When the cells are healthy, they split regularly, staying together and making the filaments longer and longer. When the spirals reach a certain length – for AlgaeLab strain, 8-9 turns – they break naturally, forming smaller spiral filaments that start to grow and lengthen themselves. If the nutrients in the culture are inadequate, the filaments can break more easily, creating many shorter strands. Also, otherwise healthy strands can be broken if there is violent motion somewhere in the culture, such as strong splashing, or intense bubbling caused by high-pressure air (not likely to be caused by aquarium pumps and bubblers), or certain kinds of water pumps. **Spirulina spirals are not difficult to break**, as they are less than one tenth of the width of human hair across, and lack any sort of tough cell wall. Inexpensive aquarium pumps, which use centrifugal force to push water around, are often dangerous to Spirulina, and in fact I have watched a little $7 pump chop my Spirulina to bits! **A lot of breakage is not good for Spirulina**, and should be avoided; it can also lead to the formation of straight filaments, which are more difficult to filter.

Measuring Culture Density

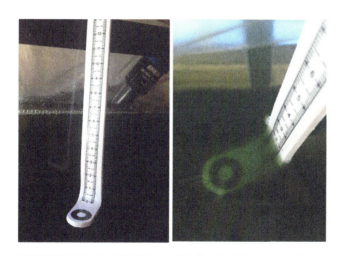

Figure 24: Commercially-obtained algae density meauring wand. You can make your own quite easily!

Culture density is expressed in terms of how far through the culture you can see a high-contrast item.[16] A handy tool to make this measurement is called a Secchi disk. A real Secchi disk is pretty big (20 cm diameter), has black and white quadrants, and is used in natural bodies of water like ponds and lakes. Since we only need to measure short distances, and our tanks are relatively small, it makes the most sense to use a mini-Secchi disk, such as the commercially-obtained one shown in Figure 24 (bought from Aquatic Eco-Systems), or by making your own. This can be done by attaching a white object (say, a piece of white plastic, or paper sealed in packing tape) about 1" diameter to the tip of a ruler, or a piece of wire with centimeter marks on it. The white object should stick out to the side of the tip, as shown in Figure 24. Then you can stick it in your tank and see at what depth it disappears from your sight. It is a surprisingly consistent and useful measurement. For example, if the depth is more than 4 cm, it's better to wait before harvesting; if it is 4 cm or less, go ahead and harvest. It is also a good way to track the growth of your culture, much better than qualitative judgements of how dense it looks! Over time, though, you will develop an "eye" for when the density is high enough...

---

16 It is also expressed in grams per liter, cells per liter, optical density, and several other ways that are a bit too technical for this book... this way is by far the simplest to measure.

Section 9: For More Information

Here are some resources I have found helpful in learning how to grow Spirulina. I hope they are helpful for you as well!

Spirulina Inspiration:

"Earth Food Spirulina: How This Remarkable Blue-Green Algae Can Transform Your Health and Our Planet", by Robert Henrikson. Ronore Enterprises, 1997.
http://www.spirulinasource.com/PDF.cfm/EarthFoodSpirulina.pdf

Also available as a paperback on Amazon.

Practical guides for growing Spirulina outdoors in tropical climates:

"A Teaching Module for the Production of Spirulina", by Antenna Technologies.
www.antenna.ch/en/documents/Modu_UK.pdf

"Grow Your Own Spirulina", by Jean-Paul Jourdan.
http://www.antenna.ch/en/documents/Jourdan_UK.pdf

Spirulina Science and Technology:

"*Spirulina platensis (Arthrospira):* Physiology, Cell-biology, and Biotechnology", edited by Avigad Vonshak. Taylor & Francis, 1997.

Available on Amazon and through Google Books.

Spirulina Nutrition Science:

"*Spirulina in Human Nutrition and Health*", edited by M.E. Gershwin and A. Belay. CRC Press, 2008.

Available on Amazon and through Google Books.

Section 10: Troubleshooting Guide

This is meant as a quick reference in case you have any questions or issues...

Issue	Possible Diagnoses/Solutions	Reference Page #s
After starting a new tank, Spirulina turn yellow/brown and clump after a day or so.	1. Wrong water source used to make medium. 2. Wrong nutrient mixes/proportions. 3. Temperature too high/low.	20 64 13, 22, 49
Culture doesn't die, but won't grow – culture stays pale green.	Inadequate light, or a lesser version of one of the above problems.	48
Culture has been growing fine for some time, suddenly (in less than 24 hours) turns yellowish & thin. Clumps appear.	1. High temperature event – turn down heater, partially shade culture from intense sunlight. 2. Low temperature event – use heater set to approx. 60F at night. 3. Problem with medium – renew medium immediately.	22, 49 22, 49 38
Culture slowly (over several days or more) becomes yellowish, clumps, does not grow.	Medium is old, or imbalanced. May have used wrong amount of Make-Up mix. Renew medium.	38
Clumps appear in the culture, floating or stuck to bubbler/heater/walls.	If minor, use strainer to remove from tank. If major, empty and clean tank, straining out all clumps. If culture thins significantly, check temperature and/or renew medium.	37
Spirulina strands are short (averaging less than 4 turns as seen in microscope), and or getting shorter. OR: harvested Spirulina is "sticky", and/or seems to be passing through the filter more than before...	Something in your system is breaking up the Spirulina colonies – a pump, strong splashing, or intense bubbling. Inadequate nutrients can also contribute to the problem. If the Spirulina have changed from curly to straight, dump the culture & start over with a healthy starter culture.	51
More jelly and algae clumps than I'd like...	Harvest more often!	37
Everything is going fine...	Fill a bottle with good culture and keep it in reserve!	17

Section 11: Fresh Spirulina Recipes

So, what do you do with your lovely blue-green creamy stuff? Although you can just eat it up directly, (perhaps flavored, see below), you'll probably want to include it in as many foods as possible, to make it as yummy as possible, and to eat as much of it as possible – the more you eat, the greater the benefits! To do this, and keep everything super-palatable, will take some creativity... The following section is meant to give you some ideas and inspiration in your culinary journey with fresh Spirulina. But feel free to add Spirulina to any food, to enhance nutrition without adding bulk!

If you come up with any cool new recipes, be sure to send them to us at contact@algaelab.org; we will post them so everyone can benefit!

Shakes & Smoothies

Pop your Spirulina into a blender with other yummy stuff and press the button! The easiest way to enjoy fresh Spirulina, other than eating it directly, is to blend it with juice; carrot juice, grapefruit juice, and orange juice all work well. The fresh stuff can be combined with almost anything – soy milk, rice milk, coconut water – since it has such a neutral taste.

But with a little more effort you can take things much further, and make smoothies that will knock your socks off with their deliciousness and energy boost. Fresh, raw fruits & veggies are already so good for you; with the spirally goodness they are even better, and much more satisfying...

You don't need to change your favorite smoothie recipe for Spirulina; just throw a tablespoon or two in; the fresh stuff won't change the flavor much. If want to develop new smoothie recipes, here are some handy-dandy charts that should help you play with the dominant flavors of each main type of smoothie.

Sweet & Tangy Fruit Shake

Sweet tangy fruity shakes are excellent in the morning, or any time you need to get moving! They offer quick energy, balanced by antioxidants to protect your body from the free radicals generated by exercise, and all the other plant compounds that support your long-term health, plus the sustaining power of Spirulina! These smoothies are great on hot days, as the electrolytes make up for those lost in sweat, and all the fruit tends to keep you cool. The vitamins and tartness can also be great for dealing with colds and other respiratory illness.

Make the shake using some combination of the ingredients in this table:

Sweetness	Tanginess/ Tartness	Creaminess	Bulk/Satisfy-ingness	Minerals, etc.
Bananas	Lemon, whole/ juice	Peanut Butter	Oatmeal – cooked, rolled, or whole	Young spinach
Pineapple	Berries	Walnuts	Flax seeds	Emergen-C/ other electro-lyte powder
Berries	Yogurt	Almonds	Chia seeds	Chia seeds
Orange juice	Rhubarb	Cashews	SPIRULINA	SPIRULINA
Dates, pitted		Avocado	Yogurt	
Pomegranate juice		Yogurt		
Carrot juice		Coconut oil/ flesh		
Coconut water				
Mango				

And two ingredients that don't fall into these categories: ginger, a strong anti-inflammatory that adds a yummy zip to any shake, and cacao nibs/powder, which adds chocolately goodness (and powerful antioxidants) without the sugar and fat of actual chocolate. The combination of ginger with lemon makes this sort of shake automatically yummy, almost no matter which other ingredients you use. Finally, I top off with water or soy/rice/almond milk, thinning out overly intense flavors and making it easier to blend.

Play with the ingredients of this matrix to get the combination of flavors that work for you and get you going!

As an example of a sweet tangy fruit smoothie, this is what I drink every morning:

Dr. Friendly's Morning Shake

- Handful Walnuts and/or almonds
- Handful Dates, Pitted
- Chunk of ginger (up to 1" cube)
- Half a whole lemon (optional, need a strong blender (Vitamix/Blendtec) for

this)
- 2 heaping tablespoons fresh spirulina
- Handful young spinach greens
- 2-4 cups frozen fruit – blueberries, peaches, strawberries, pineapple, mango, etc.
- Heaping tablespoon of yogurt (use soy yogurt for vegan)
- A splash of pomegranate juice!

Top off with water. Blend thoroughly.

Here's another one I like a lot: this is a quick one that gets me going for hikes, dance parties, or other strenuous activity:

- Handful of walnuts/almonds
- Chunk of Ginger (up to 1" cube)
- Half a whole lemon (optional, need a strong blender (Vitamix/Blendtec) for this)
- Handful young spinach greens
- 2 Heaping tablespoons fresh spirulina
- Top with carrot juice, and blend!

If you drink enough of these, you will slowly turn orange... and you'll feel great!

Comfort Food Shake

This type of shake just makes you feel warm and filled with goodness. Think sweet baked goods, or pudding, but full of superfood; it won't leave you on the couch! Fresh Spirulina really comes into its own in this shake, as the taste of powdered Spirulina would not work with the subtle, sweet flavors here... also, Spirulina helps the body to metabolize fat! If you want to add bulk and stick-to-the-ribs satisfaction to this type of shake, throw in some rolled oats.

Sweetness	Flavor/Spice	Creaminess
Bananas	Vanilla extract/beans	Peanut Butter
Coconut water	Cacao nibs/powder	Walnuts
Dates, pitted	Cinnamon	Almonds
Mango	Nutmeg	Cashews
Bee pollen	Ginger	Avocado
Blueberries		Coconut oil/flesh

Sweet Veggie Shake

This one may seem a little counter-intuitive at first, as most of you are probably used to eating your veggies in a savory context, but bear with me, this can be quite delicious if you've ever enjoyed a fresh carrot or green bean! This is a simple sort of shake, particularly nice on warm summery or springtime days, made with peas just picked from your garden... This is another shake where the neutral taste of fresh Spirulina works well.

Sweetness	Vegginess	Creaminess
Carrot juice	Fresh snap peas	Almonds
Rice milk	Fresh shelled peas	Cashews
Soy milk	Green beans	Avocado
	Carrots	SPIRULINA
	Young spinach greens	Oats/oatmeal

Savory Smoothie/Cold Soup

Pungency	Vegginess	Satisfyingness
White onion	Tomatoes	Avocado
Green onion/scallion	Cucumber	Pumpkin seeds
Garlic	Celery	Olives, pitted
Chives	Chard	SPIRULINA
Parsley	Kale	Olive oil
Lemon – whole/juice	Fresh snap peas	
Ginger	Fresh shelled peas	
Balsamic vinegar	Green beans	
Cider vinegar	Carrots	
Sea salt	Young spinach greens	

Don't imagine that smoothies must always be sweet – some of the best I've had have been savory, salty shakes of greens and veggies. Spirulina (fresh or powder) goes very well with this sort of shake, which could be considered a variation on gazpacho. In fact, if you chop instead of blend the onions and parsley, and go heavy on the tomatoes, you'll have something very much like gazpacho...

Top off with water, blend, salt to taste, and enjoy! Garnish with a little parsley to make it fancy. These are particularly delicious during hot summer afternoons...

Hot Soup

While cooking with Spirulina somewhat defeats the purpose, as many vital nutrients are broken down by the heat, adding fresh Spirulina to a soup right before serving is a great way to add super-nutrition to your tummy-warming concoctions. Try mixing Spirulina with miso soup, or adding a dollop of the fresh stuff to black bean soup, swirl it with some yogurt to make a white-blue-green yin yang... Also try it with carrot-ginger soup, minestrone, etc.

An example:

Spanish Green Soup With Fresh Spirulina!

- 1 onion, minced
- 1 clove garlic, minced
- 6 potatoes, peeled and thinly sliced
- 2 quarts cold water
- 6 ounces chorizo sausage, thinly sliced (for vegan version, substitute soy sausage)
- 2 1/2 teaspoons salt
- ground black pepper to taste
- 1 pound kale, rinsed and cut into strips (julienned)
- 2 heaping tablespoons fresh Spirulina

Directions

1. Saute onion and garlic in a few tablespoons of olive oil for 3 minutes, using a large saucepan and medium heat. Stir in potatoes and cook, stirring constantly, 3 minutes more. Pour in water, bring to a boil, and let boil gently for 20 minutes, until potatoes are mushy.
2. Meanwhile, in a large skillet over medium-low heat, cook sausage until it has released most of its fat, 10 minutes. Drain.
3. Mash potatoes or puree the potato mixture with a blender or food processor. Stir the sausage, salt and pepper into the soup and return to medium heat. Cover and simmer 5 minutes.
4. Just before serving, stir kale into soup and simmer for 5 minutes, until kale

is tender and jade green. Stir in a tablespoon of olive oil, swirl in fresh Spirulina, and serve...

Salsa and Guacamole

As guacamole is already green, it is a great way to sneak Spirulina nutrition into food that anyone would find attractive. You can add fresh Spirulina (or the powder) to your favorite guacamole recipe, or try this one:

Ultra-Green Guacamole

- 3 avocados
- 1 lime
- 1 teaspoon salt
- 1/2 cup diced onion
- 3 tablespoons fresh cilantro, chopped
- 2 roma (plum) tomatoes, diced
- 1 teaspoon minced garlic
- 2 heaping tablespoons fresh Spirulina (or 1 of the powder)
- 1 pinch ground cayenne pepper (optional)

Directions

1. Pit and peel the avocados, and put them in a mixing bowl.
2. Squeeze in the lime juice, add salt and Spirulina, and mash.
3. Mix in onion, cilantro, tomatoes, and garlic.
4. Stir in cayenne pepper.
5. Refrigerate 1 hour for best flavor, or serve immediately.

Salad Dressing

Fresh Spirulina works great in salad dressings too – it's easy to blend in and adds creaminess and nutrition. It's good to employ a little color management, though, as a salad of just greens with green dressing starts to look a little Dr. Suess-y!

Salad Dressing

- ¼ cup tahini, aka sesame butter
- 1 clove garlic
- juice of 1 lemon
- 1 tablespoon miso
- 1 tablespoon fresh Spirulina

Mix up the ingredients and dress the salad.

Ideas for colorful salads: use lots of tomatoes, cabbage, cucumbers, shredded carrots...

Pesto

Pesto, like guacamole, is a perfect opportunity to introduce more Spirulina, as it is green and creamy already; the strong taste will cover even the flavor of most powdered Spirulina...

Fresh Spirulina Pesto

- 2 cups fresh basil leaves (pack into cups to measure)
- 1/2 cup extra virgin olive oil
- 1/4 cup pine nuts (pignolis) and/or walnuts
- 3 medium-sized garlic cloves
- 2 tablespoons fresh Spirulina
- 1/2 cup grated Parmesan, Romano, or hard Pecorino cheese
- 1/3 cup chopped fresh parsley (optional)
- Salt and black pepper to taste

Directions
1. Combine basil, nuts, and garlic in a food processor, pulse until coaresly chopped.
2. Add the oil and Spirulina, and process till smooth.
3. Add salt and pepper to taste.
4. Mix in cheese and optional parsely and serve.
5. If freezing, omit cheese, Spiruina, and parsley, and use only half the oil in

food processor. Drizzle the remaining oil on top before storing. When serving, thaw and then mix in remaining ingredients...

If you come up with any recipes, ideas, tips, or tricks that you'd like to share, please send them to us at contact@algaelab.org, and we'll post them where everyone can benefit!

And, most of all, **HAVE FUN!**
Best wishes from all the AlgaeLab crew!
— Dr. Aaron Wolf Baum

Appendix A: Nutrient Mix Recipes

First, and foremost: you are producing food here, so:

*** ALWAYS USE FOOD-GRADE CHEMICALS IN YOUR NUTRIENT MIXES! ***

Some of these ingredients are most often available as "technical grade" ingredients for non-food purposes – fireworks, "stump remover", etc.; **do not use these**! Look for "food-grade" only.

Starter Mix

All measurements are in grams (or milligrams, or milliliters) per liter of fresh water.

Ingredient	Amount	Suggested Source
Sodium bicarbonate, also know as baking soda	16 g/L	Your local supermarket
Potassium Nitrate, also known as saltpeter	2 g/L	A butcher shop, or search online for food-grade; use the type intended to cure meats.
Sea Salt	1 g/L	Your local supermarket or health food store. <u>Do not use refined "table" salt.</u>
Ammonium phosphate (see note below)	0.1 g/L	Use brewer's diammonium phosphate, or "DAP".
Strong green tea (brewed and strained liquid, not the leaves!) See below for alternatives.	1 mL/L	Your local supermarket or health food store. Mix with iron sulfate before use — see below.
Iron Sulfate	10 mg/L	Use liquid sulfate iron supplement, e.g. http://www.healthwarehouse.com (use ¼ of a dropperful per liter of medium); mix with tea/chelator before use!

For measuring the green tea, the fact that 5 ml is almost exactly 1 teaspoon may be useful. As an alternative to the green tea, you can add 20 mg/L citric acid, or seven drops of lemon juice per liter. These ingredients are meant to "chelate" the iron, which keeps it available to the Spirulina.

To best achieve this chelation, **combine the chelator — green tea/citric acid/lemon juice — and the iron sulfate before putting them into the medium**. Add a tablespoon or so of water to the citric acid or lemon juice to ensure that everything dissolves completely. The green tea will turn dark purple as the iron is chelated; the citric acid solutions will turn yellow.

The ammonium phosphate can be monoammonium phosphate $(NH_4)H_2PO_4$, diammonium phosphate $(NH_4)_2HPO_4$, or monopotassium phosphate, KH_2PO_4. Brewer's diammonium phosphate, or "DAP", is generally the easiest to find in food-grade form.

Sodium nitrate can be substituted for the potassium nitrate, but then it is necessary to add 0.5 g/L of potassium sulfate so that the algae get enough potassium.

If your water is very "soft" – i.e. less than 10 mg of calcium per liter – you must add 0.1g/L of lime, calcium chloride, or plaster to the mix. To grow in distilled water, rain water, or reverse osmosis water, add 0.1 g/L magnesium sulfate, 0.5 g/L potassium sulfate, and 0.1g/L of lime, calcium chloride, or plaster to the mix.

Freshly-made medium (i.e. powder mixed with water) can be stored for 3-5 days, though it should be kept in the dark. Refrigerating it is best, though it should be warmed up before use, as sudden temperature changes can kill the algae.

Make-Up Mix

This makes enough for several months of harvesting. It is only used at harvest time.

Ingredient	Amount	Suggested Source
Potassium Nitrate, also known as saltpeter	1.4 kg	A butcher shop, or search online for food-grade; use the type intended to cure meats.
Ammonium phosphate (see note below)	50 g	Use brewer's diammonium phosphate, or "DAP".
Potassium sulfate	30 g	Use "reagent" grade chemical.
Magnesium sulfate, also known as Epsom Salt	20 g	Your local supermarket.

Since it is difficult, if not impossible, to locate food-grade potassium sulfate, use the reagent grade chemical, which is the purest form that is readily available. If the water is high in sulfates (>20 mg/L),[17] the potassium sulfate can be omitted.

If your water is particularly "soft" – i.e. lacking in minerals – add 10g of lime.

These recipes are adapted from the online pamphlet by Antenna Technologies, "A Teaching Module for the Production of Spirulina" by J. Falquet, June 1999.

---

17 This is unusual.

Appendix B: Growing Up From a Test Tube

If you cannot get a bottle of starter Spirulina culture from AlgaeLab.org, you can get a starter culture from a culture library. What you are looking for is cultures of *Arthrospira platensis*, or *Arthrospira maxima* — these are the proper scientific names of the two commercially-grown algae strains; "Spirulina" is just a nickname. Don't try to grow other strains, even if they have "Arthrospira" or "Spirulina" in their names, unless you are certain that they are safe!

In the U.S., you can get such algae samples from UTex (www.utex.org), or NCMA (ncma.bigelow.org , formerly CCMP). In Europe, CCAP (http://www.ccap.ac.uk) or SAG (http://sagdb.uni-goettingen.de) can provide live Spirulina culture. In Australia, contact the CSIRO's Australian National Algae Culture Collection (http://www.csiro.au/Organisation-Structure/National-Facilities/Australian-National-Algae-Culture-Collection.aspx), and ask for their Arthrospira maxima (strain CS-328). Most of these insititutions will ship internationally as well, so you should be able to get the live culture you need to start.

In general, you will receive only a small test tube of culture — 15 mL is typical. It will take some more time, care, and equipment to get to a large, harvestable culture, but it certainly can be done!

When the Spirulina arrive at your doorstep, they will be highly stressed do to a lack of light and variable temperatures. They will also be floating in a generic medium that is not optimized for Spirulina. Even though the medium you will be putting them in *is* optimized for Spirulina, the sudden shift of medium composition can shock them, and even kill them if it is too sudden. This means that you must handle them very carefully at first!

Once you understand how to raise up such algae samples to larger volumes, you may come up with variations on this approach. It is important, though, to have your growth system set up beforehand, so that you can start babying your spirals right away...

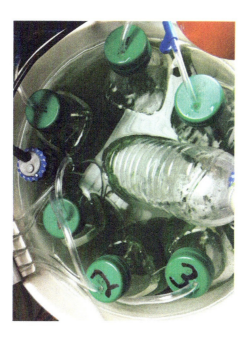

Figure 25: Growth bottles in a heat bath. In this case, the light is above the bucket (moved aside for this photo).

Equipment Needed

- A sample of live Spirulina culture (15mL is typical, more is always better...)
- 4x 250 mL soda bottles, carefully washed and rinsed
- Aquarium air pump (the smallest size - for 5-10 gallons - will do fine)
- 5' of aquarium air tubing
- 3x airline T's (three-way airline connectors)
- 4x small airstones (optional, these can help with bubbling uniformity)
- Aquarium heater (with a range up to at least 94F)
- Bucket or other water container capable of holding soda bottles and heater
- 1 bucket or other water container, capable of holding all four soda bottles and the heater (fully submerged). Clear walls are better but not required. One option is using the tank you will be growing the culture in...

- 2′ of stiff but flexible wire, such as baling wire
- Lamp or fluorescent fixture (optional if sunlight is available, see below)
- Light meter – photography or other type capable of measuring Lux level (note: many smartphones have apps that make them into light meters!) This is optional, but definitely a good idea...

Grow-Up Procedure

1. Drill two holes into each soda bottle top, just enough to pass the tubing with a little pushing (1/4″ for typical airline tubing).
2. Push a length of airline hose through one of the holes in a soda bottle top, far enough so that it pushes into the bottom of the bottle. Attach an airstone (optional), and plug the other end into the aquarium air pump, using a check valve if the pump is lower than the bottle. Cut 4″ (10 cm) of airline tubing, push it 1/4″ (0.5 cm) through the other hole, and let the rest hang down. This tube allows air to escape, and this configuration prevents microorganisms from falling into the hole if bubbling stops.
3. Set up the bucket out of direct sunshine, where the bottles inside can be illuminated by the light source. Put at least 4″ of water into the bucket, sufficient to submerge the submersible part of the heater. See Figure 25. This is called a heat bath.
4. Use the wire to create a set of loops that will keep the bottles vertical when they are floating in the heat bath (see Figure 25).
5. Set the heater to 85F (29C). This lower temperature is intended to reduce the shock to the cells, by minimizing sudden temperature changes.
6. Position the light, and measure the intensity of the light where the bottles will be. This should be no more than 2 kLux (~25 microEinsteins PAR,[18] if you have a real PAR meter). Move the light to get the right amount of light. Eventually (Step 13), you will be moving it closer to get more light on the cultures. If you are using sunlight, you may need to use thin white fabric in layers to get the right amount.
7. Make 1 liter of Spirulina medium, combining 1 liter of water (be sure to read "What Water to Use" in Section 3!), 1.5 tablespoons of Starter Mix, and 1/5 of a squeeze of the iron juice (you'll have to eyeball this, a little bit more or less won't kill your algae).
8. Fill one of your 250mL bottles ¼ of the way (~60 mL) with the medium.

---

[18] PAR = Photosynthetically Active Radiation, usually considered to be wavelengths between 400 and 700 nm. MicroEinsteins are the same as micromoles of photons per second.

Keep the remaining medium in the fridge (labelling it is a good idea!). Pour half of the culture sample into the bottle. Put the remaining half in a place that gets less than 2 kLux of light, and doesn't get too hot (>85F/29C)) or too cold (<65F/18C). Use this reserve to re-start if something goes wrong.

9. Closely examine the culture in the bottle, so that you will be able to tell when the Spirulina start growing. You may want to take a picture under repeatable lighting conditions, so that you will be better able to judge changes in its density.

10. Place the bottle in the heat bath. Make sure that the wire loops around its neck will reliably keep it upright! Plug in the air pump, and verify that the bubbling. Move the light into position so that the culture is being illuminated at 2 kLux or less.

11. Check on the temperature, light level, bubbling and culture density at least daily. It will take at least 3-5 days before it starts to thicken noticeably.

12. Once the culture starts to thicken, turn the heater up to 90F (32C). Wait 24 hours.

13. If the culture continues to grow, double the light level to 4 kLux.

14. Once the culture has a strong blue-green color and is clearly growing (this often takes a week or more), fill another soda bottle ¼ full of medium and float it in the heat bath for 15 minutes to equalize the temperature. Then add the warmed medium to the culture, returning the remaining medium to the fridge.

15. Once the half-full bottle has darkened noticeably, double it again with warmed medium, filling the bottle 7/8 full (leave some room at the top to keep culture from being pushed up through the air outlet). Increase the light level to 8 kLux.

16. Once the full bottle has darkened noticeably, prepare a second bottle, using one of the T's to run air to both bottles. Pour half of the culture into the new bottle, and top both off with warmed medium. Raise the heat bath temperature to 94F (34C). Pay close attention to the bubbling rates inside the bottles, it can easily fall out of balance. Rates can be equalized by adjusting the depth of the air outlet tube tips; putting them deeper in the heat bath water will slow the bubbling rate so that the rates can be balanced. Having an equal depth of culture in each bottle is also critical for equalizing bubbling rates.

17. Once the two bottles have darkened noticeably, prepare two more bottles, and split the two bottles into the four, topping off with warmed medium. Again, watch the balance of the bubbling rates so that all bottles are bubbled approximately equally.

18. When all four bottles are green, congratulations, you are ready to inoculate a tank!

CPSIA information can be obtained at www.ICGtesting.com
Printed in the USA
BVOW10s1023271014

372304BV00003B/13/P